C000220658

HEIGHT/WEIGHT — ADULTS (DESIRABLE)

	Height without shoes (cm)	Mean −10% (kg)	Mean for medium build (kg)	Mean +10% (kg)	Mean +20% (kg)	Height without shoes (ft in)	Mean −10% (st lb)	Mean for medium build (st lb)	Mean +10% (st lb)	Mean +20% (st lb)
Men	155	49	54	59	64	5 1	7 9	8 7	9 4	10 2
	157	50	55	61	66	5 2	7 12	8 10	9 8	10 6
	160	51	57	63	68	5 3	8 1	8 13	9 11	10 10
	162	52	58	64	69	5 4	8 3	9 2	10 1	10 13
	165	54	60	66	71	5 5	8 7	9 6	10 5	11 3
	167	55	62	68	74	5 6	8 10	9 10	10 9	11 8
	170	57	64	70	76	5 7	9 0	10 0	11 0	12 0
	172	59	65	72	78	5 8	9 4	10 4	11 4	12 4
	175	60	67	74	80	5 9	9 7	10 8	11 9	12 9
	177	63	71	78	85	5 10	10 2	10 13	12 2	13 1
	180	64	71	79	85	5 11	10 2	11 3	12 5	13 6
	183	66	74	80	88	6 0	10 6	11 8	13 0	13 11
	186	68	75	83	90	6 1	10 10	11 12	13 2	14 3
	188	70	78	85	93	6 2	10 14	12 2	13 6	14 7
	191	72	80	88	96	6 3	11 5	12 8	13 11	15 0
Women	142	40	45	49	54	4 8	6 5	7 1	7 10	8 6
	145	41	46	51	55	4 9	6 7	7 3	7 13	8 8
	147	43	47	52	56	4 10	6 10	7 6	8 2	8 12
	150	44	49	54	58	4 11	6 12	7 9	8 6	9 2
	152	45	50	55	60	5 0	7 1	7 12	8 9	9 6
	155	46	51	56	61	5 1	7 4	8 0	8 12	9 9
	157	48	53	58	63	5 2	7 7	8 5	9 2	9 13
	160	49	55	60	65	5 3	7 10	8 9	9 6	10 4
	162	51	57	63	68	5 4	8 0	8 13	9 13	11 0
	165	52	59	64	70	5 5	8 4	9 4	10 1	11 5
	167	54	61	66	72	5 6	8 7	9 7	10 6	11 10
	170	57	63	68	74	5 7	8 11	9 11	10 10	12 0
	172	58	64	70	76	5 8	9 1	10 1	11 0	12 5
	175	59	66	72	79	5 9	9 4	10 5	11 5	12 9
	177	61	68	74	81	5 10	9 8	10 9	11 9	12 10

All weights with indoor clothes, no shoes.

BODY MASS INDEX (BMI) NORMAL VALUES

Height (metres)

Weight (st/lbs)	1.36	1.44	1.52	1.60	1.68	1.76	1.84	1.92	2.00									Weight (kg)
19st 7lbs	67	63	60	57	54	51	48	46	44	42	40	38	37	35	34	32	31	124
	66	62	59	56	53	50	48	45	43	41	39	38	36	35	33	32	30	122
19st	65	61	58	55	52	49	47	45	43	41	39	37	35	34	33	31	30	120
7lbs	64	60	57	54	51	48	46	44	42	40	38	36	35	33	32	31	29	118
	63	59	56	53	50	48	45	43	41	39	37	36	34	33	31	30	29	116
18st	62	58	55	52	49	47	45	42	40	39	37	35	34	32	31	30	28	114
7lbs	61	57	54	51	48	46	44	42	40	38	36	35	33	32	30	29	28	112
	59	56	53	50	48	45	43	41	39	37	36	34	32	31	30	29	27	110
17st	58	55	52	49	47	44	42	40	38	37	35	33	32	31	29	28	27	108
7lbs	57	54	51	48	46	44	41	39	38	36	34	33	31	30	29	28	26	106
	56	53	50	47	45	43	41	39	37	35	34	32	31	29	28	27	26	104
16st	55	52	49	47	44	42	40	38	36	34	33	31	30	29	28	27	25	102
7lbs	54	51	48	46	43	41	39	37	35	34	32	31	30	28	27	26	25	100
	53	50	47	45	42	40	38	36	35	33	32	30	29	28	27	26	24	98
15st	52	49	46	44	42	39	37	36	34	32	31	30	28	27	26	25	24	96
7lbs	51	48	45	43	41	39	37	35	33	32	30	29	28	27	25	24	23	94
	49	47	44	42	40	38	36	34	33	31	30	28	27	26	25	24	23	92
14st	49	46	43	41	39	37	35	33	32	30	29	28	27	25	24	23	22	90
7lbs	48	45	42	40	38	36	34	33	31	29	28	27	26	25	24	23	22	88
	46	44	41	39	37	35	34	32	30	29	28	26	25	24	23	22	21	86
13st	45	43	41	38	36	35	33	31	30	28	27	26	25	24	23	22	21	84
7lbs	44	42	40	37	35	34	32	30	29	28	26	25	24	23	22	21	20	82
	43	41	39	37	35	33	31	30	28	27	26	25	24	23	22	21	20	80
12st	42	40	38	36	34	32	30	29	28	26	25	24	23	22	21	20	19	78
7lbs	41	39	37	35	33	31	30	28	27	26	25	23	22	21	20	19	18	76
	40	38	36	34	32	30	29	28	26	25	24	23	22	21	20	19	18	74
11st	39	37	35	33	31	30	28	27	26	24	23	22	21	20	20	19	18	72
7lbs	38	36	34	32	30	29	27	26	25	24	23	22	21	20	19	18	17	70
	37	35	33	31	29	28	27	25	24	23	22	21	20	19	18	17	17	68
10st	36	34	32	30	29	27	26	25	23	22	21	20	19	19	18	17	16	66
7lbs	35	33	31	29	28	26	25	24	23	22	21	20	19	18	17	16	15	64
	34	32	30	28	27	25	24	23	22	21	20	19	18	17	16	16	15	62
9st	32	31	29	27	26	25	23	22	21	20	19	18	17	16	16	15	15	60
7lbs	31	30	28	26	25	24	23	22	20	19	18	17	16	16	15	14	14	58
	30	29	27	26	24	23	22	21	20	19	18	17	16	15	15	14	14	56
8st	29	28	26	25	23	22	21	20	19	18	17	16	16	15	14	14	13	54
7lbs	28	27	25	24	23	21	20	19	18	17	16	16	15	14	14	13	13	52
	27	26	24	23	22	21	20	18	18	17	16	15	14	14	13	12	12	50
7st	26	24	23	22	21	20	19	18	17	16	15	14	14	13	12	12	12	48
	25	23	22	21	20	19	18	17	16	15	14	14	13	12	12	11	11	46
	24	22	21	20	19	18	17	16	15	14	14	13	12	12	11	11	11	44
6st 7lbs	23	21	20	19	18	17	16	16	15	14	13	12	12	11	11	11	10	42

	4'6"	4'9"	5'0"	5'3"	5'6"	5'9"	6'0"	6'3"	6'6"

Height (feet)

	Ideal	Overweight	Obese	Very obese
Men	20 – 25	25 – 30	30 – 40	40 +
Women	18 – 23	23 – 28	28 – 40	40 +

WEIGHT 3

INFECTIOUS DISEASES

Disease	Incubation period (days)	Quarantine period (days)	Infectivity
Acquired immune deficiency syndrome (AIDS)	3 months– 15 years		For life
Anthrax	3–7 (may be a few hours)	None	Spores — up to 15 years in soil
Botulism (ingestion)	12–36 hours or 4–14 days	None	Not applicable
Botulism (wound infection)	Few days — several months		
Brucellosis	14–30	None	Rarely from human to human
Chickenpox	11–21	21	Until last scab separates
Cholera	1–5	5	7–14 days (whilst *Vibrio cholerae* in faeces)
Diphtheria	2–7	12	2–4 weeks (until swabs free from bacilli)
Dysentery (amoebic)	21–28 (may be months)	None	Years if untreated
Dysentery (bacillary)	1–4	7	3–4 weeks untreated (until swabs negative)
Enterobiasis	14–21		During infection
Erysipelas	1–5	None	10 days if untreated
Gonorrhoea	3–9	None	Years if untreated
Hepatitis acute Type 'A'	14–42	None	Uncertain
Type 'B'	42–175		Isolation no value
	10–40	None	Up to 7 days from onset
Hepatitis C	2–20 weeks	None	Until antigen negative
Hepatitis D	4–6 weeks (probably as for hepatitis B)	None	Until antigen negative
Influenza	1–3	None	5 days after onset
Leptospirosis	6–12	None	Rarely from human to human
Measles	8–15	14	4 days before and 5 days after rash
Meningococcal meningitis	2–10	7	24 days (until nasal swabs negative)
Mononucleosis infectious	4–14	None	Not known
Mumps	12–26	28	2 days before and 9 days after swelling
Paratyphoid	1–10	Until repeated swabs negative	As long as faecal swabs positive
Plague	2–6	6	Pneumonic — during duration of disease
Poliomyelitis	7–21	21	Greatest in first few days of acute illness
Pertussis	7–14	21	7 days after exposure, 3 weeks after symptoms
Psittacosis	7–14	None	During acute illness
Rabies	14–63	None	Rarely from human to human
Relapsing fever	5–8	8	Untreated blood secretions 4–6 weeks
Rubella	14–21	10–21	4 days after catarrhal symptoms
Salmonella (food poisoning)	12–48 hours	Until repeated negative swabs	3 days to 3 weeks (very variable)
Scarlet fever	3–5	10	10 days to 3 weeks if untreated
Smallpox	10–14	14	2–3 weeks (until all scabs disappear)
Syphilis	14–112	None	2–4 years
Tetanus	4–21	None	Not from human to human
Typhoid	7–21	Until repeated swabs negative	Variable — may be 3 months or longer
Typhus (Murine)	6–14	14	Infective for lice 3 days after temperature returns to normal
Yellow fever	3–6	6	3 days after fever for mosquito

NOTIFIABLE DISEASES

Inform the Medical Officer for Environmental Health:

Acute encephalitis	Measles
Acute poliomyelitis	Meningitis
Anthrax	Meningococcal septicaemia (without meningitis)
Cholera	Mumps
Diphtheria	Ophthalma neonatorum
Dysentery (amoebic or bacillary)	Paratyphoid fever
Food poisoning (or suspected food poisoning)	Plague
Leprosy	Rabies
Leptospirosis	Relapsing fever
Malaria	Rubella

Scarlet fever	
Smallpox	
Tetanus	
Tuberculosis	
Typhoid fever	
Typhus	
Viral haemorrhagic fever	
Viral hepatitis	
Whooping cough	
Yellow fever	

Note: Reporting AIDS is voluntary — and in strict confidence — to the Director, Communicable Disease Surveillance Centre, 61 Colindale Avenue, London NW9 5EQ. Tel: 0181 200 6868.

IMMUNIZATION FOR INTERNATIONAL TRAVEL

Vaccine	Minimum age	Course	Booster interval
BCG	Birth	0.1 ml id (0.05 ml <3 months)	In high risk only — 10 yearly if skin test negative
Cholera (killed)		Killed injectable vaccine currently unavailable; oral vaccines not yet available in UK	
Diphtheria Adult booster (toxoid)		0.5 ml sc low dose vaccine OR 0.1 ml sc children's monovalent vaccine OR 0.5 ml sc Diftavax	10–20 years 0.1 ml sc
Hepatitis A gamma globulin (passive)	Rarely indicated in children	2 ml im for travel lasting <2 months 5 ml im for travel lasting 3–5 months	5 ml im
Hepatitis A vaccines			
Havrix Junior Monodose	1 year	0.5 ml im day 1 6–12 months	10 years 0.5 ml im
Havrix Monodose	16 years	1 ml im day 1 6–12 months	10 years 1 ml im
Avaxim	16 years	0.5 ml im day 1 6 months	10 years 0.5 ml im
Hep A and Hep B combined vaccine Twinrix adult	16 years	1 ml im, never iv day 1 1 month 6 months	5 years
Hepatitis B (genetically derived)	Within a few hours of birth	1 ml im day 1 1 month 6 months <12 yrs 0.5 ml im	3–5 years
Japanese B encephalitis (killed)	1 year	1 ml sc/im day 1 7–14 days 28 days for full protection	2 years 1 ml sc
Meningococcal meningitis (killed)	18 months	0.5 ml sc/im	>2 years, boost at 3 years (Mengivac) 5 years (AC Vax) <2 years boost at 1 yr 0.5 ml sc/im
Polio (live)	6 weeks	3 drops po day 1 1 month 2 months	10 years 3 drops po 5 years if travelling to high risk area
Rabies (killed)	All ages	1 ml sc/im day 1 7 days 28 days OR 0.1 ml id day 1 7 days 28 days	3 years 1 ml sc/im OR 0.1 ml id
Tetanus (toxoid)	2 months	0.5 ml sc/im day 1 1 month 2 months	1st: 10 years 0.5 ml sc/im 2nd: 10 years 0.5 ml sc/im
Tick-borne* encephalitis (killed)	All ages	0.5 ml im day 1 2–12 weeks 6–9 months	3 years 0.5 ml im

IMMUNIZATION FOR INTERNATIONAL TRAVEL (cont'd)

Vaccine	Minimum age	Course	Booster interval
Typhoid (whole cell killed)	1 year	0.5 ml sc/im day 1 0.1 ml id 4–6 weeks	3 years 0.1 ml id
Typhoid VI antigen (killed)	18 months	0.5 ml sc/im	3 years 0.5 ml sc/im
Typhoid TY21A oral (live)	6 years	1 capsule day 1 day 3 day 5	3 years, 3 dose course 1 year if living in endemic area
Yellow Fever (live)	9 months	0.5 ml sc	10 years 0.5 ml sc

*Transmitted by insect vector, minimize exposure risk.
C/I: Live vaccines in immunosuppression, pregnancy, malignant disorders.
S/P: Rapid dose schedules may not provide full cover. Don't give immunoglobulin and live vaccine at the same time. Give live vaccines on same day or 3 weeks apart (except OPV and oral typhoid which must be separate).
Advice to medical professionals available from Communicable Disease Surveillance Centre — (0171) 200 6868

DOSES OF PROPHYLACTIC ANTIMALARIAL DRUGS FOR ADULTS*

Generic name(s)	Trade names	Usual amount per tablet	Dose for chemoprophylaxis
Chloroquine	Nivaquine, Avloclor	150 mg (base)	2 tablets weekly
Proguanil	Paludrine	100 mg	2 tablets daily
Mefloquine	Lariam	250 mg (228 mg in the USA)	1 tablet weekly
Dapsone + pyrimethamine	Maloprim	100 mg + 12.5 mg	1 tablet weekly
Doxycycline	Vibramycin,[†] Nordox[†]	100 mg	1 tablet daily

*See details, including important contraindications and adverse reactions.
[†]Not licensed for this purpose.
HMSO 1995 Health Information for Overseas Travel, pp. 74, 76 (Crown copyright is reproduced with the permission of the Controller of Her Majesty's Stationery Office)

OBSTETRICAL TABLE

The normal (left) month is the first day of the last menstrual period; the bold month is the expected date of confinement. Days 1–31 of the menstrual-period month are shown in the upper line of each pair; the expected delivery day is shown in the lower (bold) line. The month at the right indicates the month into which the later dates fall.

LMP month	1	2	3	4	5	6	7	8	9	10	11	12	13	14	15	16	17	18	19	20	21	22	23	24	25	26	27	28	29	30	31	Due month
January / **October**	8	9	10	11	12	13	14	15	16	17	18	19	20	21	22	23	24	25	26	27	28	29	30	31	1	2	3	4	5	6	7	January / **November**
February / **November**	8	9	10	11	12	13	14	15	16	17	18	19	20	21	22	23	24	25	26	27	28	29	30	1	2	3	4	5	—	—	—	February / **December**
March / **December**	6	7	8	9	10	11	12	13	14	15	16	17	18	19	20	21	22	23	24	25	26	27	28	29	30	31	1	2	3	4	5	March / **January**
April / **January**	6	7	8	9	10	11	12	13	14	15	16	17	18	19	20	21	22	23	24	25	26	27	28	29	30	31	1	2	3	4	—	April / **February**
May / **February**	5	6	7	8	9	10	11	12	13	14	15	16	17	18	19	20	21	22	23	24	25	26	27	28	1	2	3	4	5	6	7	May / **March**
June / **March**	8	9	10	11	12	13	14	15	16	17	18	19	20	21	22	23	24	25	26	27	28	29	30	31	1	2	3	4	5	6	—	June / **April**
July / **April**	7	8	9	10	11	12	13	14	15	16	17	18	19	20	21	22	23	24	25	26	27	28	29	30	1	2	3	4	5	6	7	July / **May**
August / **May**	8	9	10	11	12	13	14	15	16	17	18	19	20	21	22	23	24	25	26	27	28	29	30	31	1	2	3	4	5	6	7	August / **June**
September / **June**	8	9	10	11	12	13	14	15	16	17	18	19	20	21	22	23	24	25	26	27	28	29	30	1	2	3	4	5	6	7	—	September / **July**
October / **July**	8	9	10	11	12	13	14	15	16	17	18	19	20	21	22	23	24	25	26	27	28	29	30	31	1	2	3	4	5	6	7	October / **August**
November / **August**	8	9	10	11	12	13	14	15	16	17	18	19	20	21	22	23	24	25	26	27	28	29	30	31	1	2	3	4	5	6	—	November / **September**
December / **September**	7	8	9	10	11	12	13	14	15	16	17	18	19	20	21	22	23	24	25	26	27	28	29	30	1	2	3	4	5	6	7	December / **October**

FREQUENCY OF PRESENTATIONS

Cranial — 96.0%	Breech — 3.5%	Others — 0.5%

DEVELOPMENT OF UTERUS DURING PREGNANCY

Weeks	Level of fundus
12	Above pubic symphysis
16	Halfway between symphysis and umbilicus
20	2 fingers breadth below umbilicus
24	At umbilicus
28	3 fingers breadth above umbilicus
32	Halfway between umbilicus and xiphisternum
36	At xiphisternum
40	Various levels between 32nd and 36th week ('dropping' — 14 days before term in primigravida, less in multipara, but may not occur until labour)

INVOLUTION OF UTERUS AFTER DELIVERY

Day	Height above pubis (cm)	Day	Height above pubis (cm)
1	11.0	5	9.0
2	13.5	6	8.0
3	11.0	7	7.5
4	10.0		

WEIGHT CHANGES DURING PREGNANCY (AVERAGE)

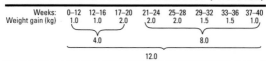

Weeks:	0–12	12–16	17–20	21–24	25–28	29–32	33–36	37–40
Weight gain (kg)	1.0	1.0	2.0	2.0	2.0	1.5	1.5	1.0

4.0   8.0

12.0

Average net loss at delivery: 8.0 kg.
Average net gain: 4.0 kg.

DISTRIBUTION OF WEIGHT GAIN AT 40 WEEKS' GESTATION (g)

	Total	Water	Fat	Protein	Other
Fetal (approx. 5.0 kg)					
Fetus	3300	2335	460	435	70
Placenta	700	590	4.5	100	5.5
Liquor	800	790	0.5	5	4.5
Mother (approx. 7.0 kg)					
Uterus	900	740	3.5	150	6.5
Breasts	400	300	12.0	80	8.0
Blood	1200	1080	19.5	130	5.5
ECF	1200	1165	—	—	—
Fat	3500	—	3500	0	0
Total	12 000	7000	4000	900	100

BLOOD CHANGES IN PREGNANCY

	Non-pregnant	34 weeks	Increment
Total blood volume (ml)	4000	5750	1750
Plasma volume (ml)	2500	4000	1500
Red cell volume (ml)	1500	1750	250
Haematocrit (whole body) (%)	37.5	30.5	—
Haematocrit (venous) (%)	40	34	—
Haemoglobin (venous)	14 g/100 ml	12 g/100 ml	—
Total haemoglobin (g)	492	597	100
Total iron (g)	1668	2000	332

PLASMA PROTEIN CHANGES IN PREGNANCY

	Non-pregnant	Term
Total (g/100 ml)	7	6
Albumin (g/100 ml)	4	3
Globulin (g/100 ml)	2.5	2.5
Fibrinogen (g/100 ml)	0.25	0.4
Total protein (g)	175	215

SEMEN (NORMAL SPERM COUNT)

Volume	3–5 ml
pH	7.4
Count	60 000 000–200 000 000/ml
Motility	90% after 45 min, 65% after 3 h
Abnormal forms	10–20%

HEIGHT/WEIGHT — CHILDREN (DESIRABLE) CENTILE CHART

Age	Weight (kg)			Height to nearest centimetre (cm)*		
	3	50	97	3	50	97
Boys						
Birth	2.5	3.5	4.4	—	50	—
3 months	4.4	5.7	7.2	55	60	65
6 months	6.2	7.8	9.8	62	66.5	71
9 months	7.6	9.3	11.6	66.5	71	76
12 months	8.4	10.3	12.8	70	75	80
18 months	9.4	11.7	14.2	75	81	87
2 years	10.2	12.7	15.7	80	87	93
3 years	11.6	14.7	17.8	86	95	102
4 years	13	15	21	94	101	110
5 years	14	19	23	100	108	117
6 years	16	21	27	105	114	124
7 years	17	23	30	110	120	130
8 years	19	25	34	115	126	137
9 years	21	27.5	39	120	132	143
10 years	23	30	44	125	137	148
11 years	25	34	50	129	142	154
12 years	27	38	58	133	147	160
13 years	30	43	64	138	153	168
14 years	33	49	71	144	160	176
15 years	39	55	76	152	167	182
16 years	46	60	79	158	172	185
17 years	49	62	80	162	174	187
18 years	50	64	82	162	175	187
Girls						
Birth	2.5	3.5	4.4	—	50	—
3 months	4.2	5.2	7.0	55	58	62
6 months	5.9	7.3	9.4	61	65	69
9 months	7.0	8.7	10.9	65	70	74
12 months	7.6	9.6	12.0	69	74	78
18 months	8.8	10.9	13.6	75	80	85
2 years	9.6	12.0	14.9	79	85	91
3 years	11.2	14.1	17.4	86	93	100
4 years	13	16	20	92	100	109
5 years	15	18	23	98	107	116
6 years	16	20	27	104	114	123
7 years	18	23	30	109	120	130
8 years	19	25	35	114	125	136
9 years	21	28	40	120	130	142
10 years	23	31	48	125	136	148
11 years	25	35	56	130	143	155
12 years	28	40	64	135	149	164
13 years	32	46	70	142	156	168
14 years	37	51	73	148	160	172
15 years	42	54	74	150	162	173
16 years	45	56	75	151	162	174
17 years	46	56	75	—	—	—
18 years	46	57	75	—	—	—

*Data are provided for the 3rd, 50th and 97th centile for each parameter. From Tanner, J. M., Whitehouse, R. H. and Takaishi, M. *Arch. Dis. Childhood* (1966), **41**, 454: adapted from West (ed.), *Neurosurg. Psychiat.*, (1956), **19**, 52.

TOOTH DEVELOPMENT

Tooth	Tooth germ fully formed	Calcification begins	Calcification of crown complete	Appearance in mouth cavity	Root complete
Deciduous					
Incisors	17th week fetal life	4 months fetal life	2–3 months	6–9 months	1–1.5 years after appearance in mouth cavity
Canines	18th week fetal life	5 months fetal life	9 months	16–18 months	
1st Molars	19th week fetal life	6 months fetal life	6 months	12–14 months	
2nd Molars	19th week fetal life	6 months fetal life	12 months	20–30 months	
Permanent					
Incisors	30th week fetal life	3–4 months (upper lateral incisor 10–12 months)	4–5 years	Lower 6–8 years Upper 7–9 years	2–3 years after appearance in mouth cavity
Canines	30th week fetal life	4–5 months	6–7 years	Lower 9–10 years Upper 11–12 years	
Premolars	30th week fetal life	1.5–2.5 years	5–7 years	10–12 years	
1st Molars	24th week fetal life	Birth	2.5–3 years	6–7 years	
2nd Molars	6th month	2.5–3 years	7–8 years	11–13 years	
3rd Molars	6th year	7–10 years	12–16 years	17–21 years	

Reproduced by kind permission from: *A Paediatric Vade-Mecum*, 7th edn Edited by B. S. B. Wood. London: Lloyd-Luke Medical Books

SUPPLEMENTAL FLUORIDE DOSAGE SCHEDULE

	Concentration of fluoride in drinking water		
	<0.3 ppm	0.3–0.7 ppm	>0.7 ppm
6 months to 2 years	0.25 mg F⁻/day	0	0
2–4 years	0.50 mg F⁻/day	0.25 mg F⁻/day	0
4–16 years	1.0 mg F⁻/day	0.50 mg F⁻/day	0

2.2 mg Sodium fluoride contains 1 mg Fluoride. F⁻ refers to the amount of fluoride ion given as a supplement.
Systemic fluoride supplements should not be given without reference to the fluoride content of the local water supply. Too much can be harmful and may cause mottling of teeth.

DRUG DOSES FOR INFANTS AND CHILDREN

Age	Weight		Body surface area (m²)	Percentage of adult dose
	kg	lb		
Birth	3.2	7	0.21	12.5
2 months	4.5	10	0.26	15
4 months	6.5	14	0.34	20
12 months	10	22	0.42	25
18 months	11	24	0.50	30
5 years	18	40	0.68	40
7 years	23	50	0.85	50
10 years	30	66	1.00	60
12 years	40	88	1.28	75
16 years	54	120	1.70	90

PROGRAMME OF IMMUNIZATION

Age	Protection against	Abbreviation	Route
2 months	Polio		By mouth
	Haemophilus b	Hib	One injection
	Diphtheria	DPT	
	Whooping cough		One injection
	Tetanus		
3 months	Polio		By mouth
	Haemophilus b	Hib	One injection
	Diphtheria	DPT	
	Whooping cough		One injection
	Tetanus		
4 months	Polio		By mouth
	Haemophilus b	Hib	One injection
	Diphtheria	DPT	
	Whooping cough		One injection
	Tetanus		
12–15 months	Measles	MMR	
	Mumps		One injection
	Rubella		
3–5 years around school entry	Measles	MMR	
	Mumps		One injection
	Rubella		
	Diphtheria	DT	One injection
	Tetanus		
	Polio		By mouth
10–13	Tuberculosis	BCG	Skin test plus injection if needed
14–19 years	Diphtheria	DT	One injection
	Tetanus		
	Polio		By mouth

IMMUNIZATION SCHEDULE

Children should receive the following vaccines:
   By 6 months: three doses of DTP, Hib and polio
   By 15 months: measles/mumps/rubella
   By school entry: fourth DT and polio; second dose measles/mumps/
      rubella
   Between 10 and 14 years: BCG
   Before leaving school: fifth polio and tetanus diphtheria (Td)

Adults should receive the following vaccines:
   Women seronegative for rubella: rubella
   Previously unimmunized subjects: polio, tetanus, diphtheria
   Subjects in high risk groups: hepatitis B, hepatitis A, influenza,
      pneumococcal vaccine

HMSO 1996 Immunisation against Infectious Diseases, p46 (Crown copyright is reproduced with the permission of the Controller of Her Majesty's Stationery Office)

VACCINES

Live vaccines	Inactivated vaccines
Measles ⎫	Diphtheria toxoid ⎫ and combination
Mumps ⎬ and MMR	Tetanus toxoid ⎬ vaccines
Rubella ⎭	Pertussis ⎭
Oral poliomyelitis	Poliomyelitis (injectable)
Oral typhoid	Haemophilus influenzae b (Hib)
BCG (TB)	Influenza
Yellow fever	Hepatitis A
	Typhoid injectable
	Meningococcal meningitis
	Japanese encephalitis
	Tick-borne encephalitis
	Hepatitis B
	Rabies
	Cholera

DOSES OF PROPHYLACTIC ANTIMALARIAL DRUGS FOR CHILDREN* (IN TABLETS)

Age:	0–5 weeks	6 weeks–11 months	1–5 years	6–11 years	>12 years
Weight:			10–19 kg	20–39 kg	>40 kg
Chloroquine (as base) weekly	37.5 mg (3.75 ml syrup)	75 mg (7.5 ml syrup)	150 mg (15 ml syrup or 1 tablet)	225 mg (22.5 ml syrup or 1½ tablets)	Adult
Proguanil daily	25 mg (¼ tablet)	50 mg (½ tablet)	100 mg (1 tablet)	150 mg (1½ tablets)	Adult
Mefloquine weekly	NR	NR	NR <15 kg 2–5 years: 62.5 mg (¼ tablet)	6–8 years 125 mg (½ tablet) 9–11 years (up to 45 kg): 187.5 mg (¾ tablet)	Adult
Maloprim weekly	NR	⅛ tablet	¼ tablet	½ tablet	Adult

*See details, including contraindications.
HMSO 1995 Health Information for Overseas Travel, pp. 76 (Crown copyright is reproduced with the permission of the Controller of Her Majesty's Stationery Office)

HAEMATOLOGY

Test		Reference range	Units	Sarstedt tube*
Blood count laboratory				
Hb	Haemoglobin	Male 12.5–18.0	g/dl	●
		Female 11.5–16.0	g/dl	●
RBC	Red blood cell count	Male 4.50–6.00	10^{12}/l	●
		Female 3.60–5.60	10^{12}/l	●
HCT	Haematocrit/ packed cell volume	Male 37.0–54.0% Female 33.0–47.0%		●
MCV	Mean cell volume	80.0–100.0	fl	●
MCH	Mean cell haemoglobin	28.0–33.0	pg	●
MCHC	Mean cell haemoglobin concentration	33.0–36.0	g/dl	●
RDW	Red cell distribution width	11.0–15.0%		●
PLTS	Platelets	150–400	10^9/l	●
MPV	Mean platelet volume	7.0–11.0	fl	●
WBC	White blood cell count	3.5–11.0	10^9/l	●
NEUT	Neutrophils	2.0–7.5	10^9/l	●
LYMPH	Lymphocytes	1.0–3.5	10^9/l	●
MONO	Monocytes	0.2–0.8	10^9/l	●
EOSIN	Eosinophils	0.0–0.4	10^9/l	●
BASO	Basophils	0.0–0.2	10^9/l	●
Retics	Reticulocytes	10–220	10^9/l	●
Sickledex haemoglobin S screen		Negative	—	●
Haemoglobin H inclusions		Negative	—	●
Heinz bodies		Negative	—	●
Malarial parasites		None demonstrated	—	●
Neutrophil alkaline phosphatase		15–100	units/ 100 neutrophils	●
ZPP (Iron deficiency screen)		15–55	µmol/mol	●
Erythrocyte sedimentation rate (ESR)		Male <10 Female <20	mm in 1 hour	○ ○
GFST	Glandular fever slide test	Negative	—	■
Haptoglobins		100–300	mg/dl	■
Plasma viscosity		1.50–1.72	cp	■
HAMS and sucrose lysis tests		Negative	—	□
Coagulation laboratory				
Clotting screen—PT and APTT		See relevant sections		▲
INR (Warfarin therapy only)		—	—	▲
PT	Prothrombin time	10.6–14.9	s	▲
APTT	Activated partial Thromboplastin time	23.0–35.0 Heparin therapy range 1.8–3.3 times normal control	s	▲ ▲
D-Dimers		<0.25	µg/ml	▲
Fibrinogen		1.5–3.8	g/l	▲
Thrombin time		10.5–15.5	s	▲
Bleeding time		2.5–9.5	min	△
Pro-coagulant factor assay		—	—	▲
Fibrinolytic investigations		—	—	△
Reptilase time		13.0–19.0	s	▲
Russell's viper venom time		—	—	△
Anti-phospholipid screen		—	—	▲
Lupus anticoagulant screen		—	—	▲
Platelet aggregation studies		—	—	△
Thrombophilia screen		—	—	▲

HAEMATOLOGY (cont'd)

Test	Reference range	Units	Sarstedt tube*
Cytology laboratory			
Film report	—	—	●
and/or WBC differential	See FBC	See FBC	●
Bone marrow examination	—	—	△
Cell marker studies	—	—	△
Specials laboratory			
Vit B$_{12}$ — serum	130–770	ng/l	■
Folate — serum	1.5–10.0	µg/l	■
Folate — red cell	95–570	µg/l	●
G.6.P.D.	3.3–5.7	iu/gHb	●
PK pyruvate kinase	5.7–10.9	iu/gHb	●
Haemoglobin electrophoresis	—	—	●
Haemoglobin A2	2.2–3.3	%totalHb	●
Haemoglobin F	Adult <0.9	%totalHb	●
	ANC female 0.5–1.1		
Methaemoglobin	0.01–0.5	g/dl	●
Osmotic fragility —	Preincubation		
	4.00–4.45	g/NaCl	□
Mean cell fragility	Postincubation		
	4.65–5.90	g/NaCl	□
Whole blood volume			
— Red cell mass	Male 25–35	ml/kg —	
	Female 20–30	body wt.	△
— Plasma volume	40–50	ml/kg —	
		body wt.	△

●, EDTA; ○, ESR tube; ■, plain/serum; □, Li hepatin; ▲, citrate; △, special tube (contact lab.).
Haematology and Blood Normal Values tables reproduced with permission from Professor Forster, Royal Liverpool University

BLOOD NORMAL VALUES

Analyte	Reference/therapeutic range	Units	Sarstedt tube*
α_1-Acid glycoprotein	0.55–1.40	g/l	□
α_1-Antitrypsin (α_1-AT)	1.1–2.3	g/l	□
α_1-Antitrypsin phenotype			■
α_2-Macroglobulin	0.7–2.4	g/l	□
ACE (angiotensin converting enzyme)	Male 18–66 Female 13–54	U/L	■
Acetylcholinesterase electrophoresis (liquor)			■
Acid phosphatase (prostate-specific)	<2.1	IU/l	■
Acid phosphatase (total)	Male <5.0 Female <4.2	IU/l	■
ACTH	09:00h 2.0–11.3	pmol/l	●
AFP (alphafetoprotein)	<2.5	MOM	■
AFP (liquor)		mg/l	■
AFP (tumour marker)	<7.0	µg/l	■
Albumin	36–52	g/l	□
Alcohol	None	mmol/l	●
Aldolase	<7.6	U/l	□

BLOOD NORMAL VALUES (cont'd)

Analyte	Reference/therapeutic range	Units	Sarstedt tube*
Aldosterone	Supine 80–300 Upright 140–850	pmol/l	☐
ALP (Alkaline phosphatase)	35–125	U/l	☐
ALP isoenzymes			☐
ALT (alanine aminotransferase)	<35	U/l	☐
Aluminium	<1.0	µmol/l	■
Amino acids			☐
Amiodarone	0.5–2.0	mg/l	■
Ammonia	10–47	µmol/l	☐
Amylase	<200	U/l	☐
Androstenedione	3–10	nmol/l	■
Anion gap	10–18	mmol/l	☐
Apo AI	>130	mg/dl	■
Apo B	75–125	mg/dl	■
Apo E phenotype			■
Arginine vasopressin (ADH)	1.0–4.5	pmol/l	■
AST (Aspartate aminotransferase)	<45	U/l	☐
β-Carotene	0.2–1.4	µmol/l	■
β$_2$-Microglobulin	<2.4	mg/l	■
Barbiturates (screen)	Not detected		■
Benzodiazepine (screen)	Not detected		■
Bicarbonate	20–30	mmol/l	☐
Bilirubin (direct)	1–6	µmol/l	☐
Bilirubin (total)	2–17	µnol/l	☐
Bilirubin —			■
Blood sugar series			☐
Bone studies			■
C-Amp	10–34.8	nmol/l	●
C-Peptide	165–993	pmol/l	■
C-Peptide/insulin ratio	5–10		■
Cadmium (whole blood)	<27	nmol/l	☐
Caeruloplasmin	Male 0.18–0.34 Female 0.14–0.46	g/l	☐
Caffeine	<258	µmol/l	☐
Calcitonin	<27	pmol/l	■
Calcium	2.20–2.60	mmol/l	☐
Calcium (adjusted)	2.20–2.60	mmol/l	☐
Calcium (ionised)	1.15–1.30	mmol/l	☐
Calcium profile			☐
CAM 17.1	<39	U/l	■
Carbamazepine	15–50	µmol/l	☐
Carboxy-haemoglobin	Non-smokers <2 Smokers <10	%	△
Cardiac enzymes			☐
Catecholamines			☐
Noradrenaline	Rested 0.5–3.0	nmol/l	☐
Adrenaline	Rested 0.1–0.3	nmol/l	☐
Dopamine	Rested <0.1	nmol/l	☐
CEA (carcinoembryonic antigen)	<4	µg/l	■
Chloride	99–109	mmol/l	☐
Cholinesterase (pseudo)	620–1370	IU/l	☐
Chromium	<5	nmol/l	△
Chromium (whole blood)	<20	nmol/l	☐
CK (creatine kinase)	Male 33–194 Female 35–143	U/l	☐
CK isoenzyme (CK-MB)	<3% <12 U/l	% and U/l	☐

BLOOD NORMAL VALUES (cont'd)

Analyte	Reference/therapeutic range	Units	Sarstedt tube*
Clonidine Stimulation test			■
Combined pituitary function test (CPFT)			■
Common alpha subunit (TSH, HCG, LH, FSH)	<1.9	µg/l	■
Copper	12.0–25.0	µmol/l	■
Cortisol	09:00h 140–500	nmol/l	■
	24:00h 50–300		
Creatinine	50–130	µmol/l	□
Creatinine clearance	85–140	ml/min	□
CRP (C-reactive protein)	<5	mg/l	□
Cyclosporin A	HPLC equiv 180–350	µg/l	□
(Whole blood)	CyA mono 200–400	µg/l	□
	CyA poly 400–1000	µg/l	□
Deoxycortisol	<30	nmol/l	■
Dexamethasone suppression test (long or overnight)			■
DHEAS	<12	µmol/l	■
Digoxin	1.0–2.5	nmol/l	□
Down's syndrome screen risk calculation			■
Erythropoietin	<50	U/l	■
Ferritin	Male 19–300	µg/l	□
	Female 17–165		
Fructosamine	<285	µmol/l	□
ESH	See additional information		□
γ-Glutamyl transferase (GGT)	Male <50	U/l	□
	Female <35		
Gastrin	10–90	ng/l	□
Globulin	22–32	g/l	□
Glucagon	0–100	pmol/l	■
Glucose	3.5–5.5 (fasting)	mmol/l	
Glucose (CSF)		mmol/l	
Glucose tolerance test (GTT)			
Glutathione peroxidase	77–126	U/g Hb	□
Glycated haemoglobin (Haemoglobin A$_{1c}$)	Non-diabetic 4.0–6.0	%	
	Adequate control 6.0–8.0	%	
	Poor control >8.0	%	
Gonadotrophin releasing hormone test GnRH test)			■
Growth hormone (GH)		mU/l	■
GTT of growth hormone suppressibility			■
Gut hormone profile			△
Haptoglobin	0.3–2.1	g/l	□
HCG-β	<10	U/l	■
Hydroxyprogesterone- (17α)	Adult <12	nmol/l	□
	Full term newborn, >48 hrs old <20		
Infertility screen–female			■
Infertility screen–male			■
Insulin		mU/l	■
Insulin/glucose ratio	>4.5–indicative of insulinoma (glu<2.2)	<14 days	■
Insulin autoantibodies			■
Insulin tolerance test (ITT)			■
Insulin-like growth factor-1 (IGF-1)	10–50	nmol/l	■
Interleukin-6	<12.5	pg/ml	■

BLOOD NORMAL VALUES (cont'd)

Analyte	Reference/therapeutic range	Units	Sarstedt tube*
Iron studies			
Iron	13–32	µmol/l	□
Iron binding capacity	45–70	µmol/l	□
% Saturation	20–55	%	□
ITT of growth hormone reserve			■
Ketones	Not detected		□
L-DOPA	0.3–1.6	mg/l	□
	1.5–8.0	µmol/l	□
Lactate	0.5–2.2	mmol/l	
Lamotrigine	4–16	µmol/l	■
LDH	<450	U/l	□
LDH (isoenzymes)		%	□
Lead (whole blood)	<0.5	µmol/l	●
LH	See additional information	U/l	■
Lipid profile			□
Cholesterol	<5.2	mmol/l	□
Triglycerides	<2.3	mmol/l	□
HDL-cholesterol	>1.0	mmol/l	□
Lipid subfractions		mmol/l	■
Lipoprotein (a) (Lp (a))	<25	mg/dl	■
Lithium	0.5–1.2	mmol/l	■
Liver profile			□
Magnesium	0.75–1.00	mmol/l	□
Magnesium (red cell)	1.7–2.6	mmol/l	□
Manganese	4–23	nmol/l	■
Manganese (whole blood)	73–210	nmol/l	●
Menopause screen			■
Mercury (whole blood)	<32	nmol/l	□
Metoclopromide test of prolactin reserve			■
Nutritional assessment			■
Oestradiol-17B	See additional information	pmol/l	■
Osmolality	288–298	mosmol/kg H_2O	□
Osteocalcin	3.2–9.7	µg/l	●
Paracetamol	<40	µmol/l	□
Pentagastrin stimulation test			■
Phenobarbitone	65–170	µmol/l	■
Phenytoin	40–80	µmol/l	■
Phosphate	0.70–1.40	mmol/l	□
Potassium	3.5–5.0	mmol/l	□
Prealbumin	0.15–0.4	g/l	□
PSA	40–49 yrs	0–2.5 ng/ml	■
(Prostatic	50–59 yrs	0–3.5 ng/ml	
specific	60–69 yrs	0–4.5 ng/ml	
antigen)	70–79 yrs	0–6.5 ng/ml	
Progesterone	>35	nmol/l	■
Prolactin	Male <350	mU/l	■
	Female <500		
Protein (CSF)	0.15–0.45	g/l	■
Protein (total)	60–80	g/l	□
Protein electrophoresis			■
Protein selectivity ratio (transferrin/IgG)	<0.2		□
Protein studies			■
PTH (intact)	1.1–6.9	pmol/l	■
PTH-Rp	<0.7–2.6	pmol/l	△
Renin (PRA)	Supine 0.2–2.8	ng/ml/h	●
	Upright 1.5–5.7		●
Reverse T3	0.14–0.54	nmol/l	■
Salicylate	<70	µmol/l	□

BLOOD NORMAL VALUES (cont'd)

Analyte	Reference/therapeutic range	Units	Sarstedt tube*
Selenium	0.7–1.6	μmol/l	□
Selenium (whole blood)	0.6–1.5	μmol/l	□
SHBG (sex hormone binding globulin)	Male 9–64	nmol/l	□
Silicon	<10	μmol/l	□
	Non-pregnant 32–96		
	Pregnant 200–380		
Sodium	135–145	mmol/l	□
Synacthen test			
Testosterone	Male 9–40	nmol/l	■
	Female <3.5		
Theophylline	55–110	μmol/l	□
Thiamine (vit B1), (red cell)	165–286	nmol/l rbc	□
Thyroid function tests (TFT)			
TSH	0.17–3.2	mU/l	■
Total T4	70–155	nmol/l	■
Free T4	11–22	pmol/l	■
Total T3	<65 yrs 1.1–2.6	nmol/l	■
	>65 yrs 0.8–2.3		
TBG (thyroxine binding globulin)	16–28	mg/l	■
TRAb (thyroid receptor antibodies)	<8	% inhibition	■
Thyroglobulin	<5	μg/l	■
Thyrotrophin releasing hormone test (TRH test)			
TRH test of prolactin reserve			
Transferrin	2.2–4.0	g/l	■
Tricyclics (screen)	Not detected		■
U & E			
Urea	2.5–7.0	mmol/l	□
Uric acid	Male 200–420	μmol/l	□
	Female 140–340*		
Valproate	350–700	μmol/l	■
Vitamin A	Newborn 1.2–2.6	μmol/l	■
	Child 1.1–2.8		
	Adult 1.1–2.3		
Vitamin C (leucocyte)	119–301	nmol/10^8 wbc	▽
(1,25-dihydroxy)	43–144	pmol/l	■
Vitamin D2 & D3			
Vitamin D2 (25-hydroxy)	<10	μg/l	■
Vitamin D3 (25-hydroxy)	Summer 10–60	μg/l	■
	Winter 5–25	μg/l	■
Vitamin E	11.6–46.5	μmol/l	■
Water deprivation test			
Zinc	12.7–20.2	μmol/l	■
Immunoglobulin analysis			
IgG	5.0–14.0*	g/l	■
IgA	1.0–4.0*	g/l	■
IgM	0.5–2.0*	g/l	■
IgG subclasses	See report	g/l	■
(IgG1–IgG4)			
IgE – total	0–1 year	<10	kU/l	■
	1–15 years	<30	kU/l	■
	over 15 years	<100	kU/l	■
Allergen specific	<0.35*	kU/l	■

●, EDTA; ○, ESR tube; ■, plain/serum; □, Li heparin; ▲, citrate; △, special tube (contact lab.).

CEREBROSPINAL FLUID VALUES

	Units	Premature	Newborn	Child	Adolescent	Adult
Appearance:				Clear and colourless ─────		
Cells						
Polymorphs	no./l	$0\text{–}100 \times 10^6$	$0\text{–}70 \times 10^6$	0	0	0
	(no./mm³)	(0–100)	(0–70)	(0)	(0)	(0)
Lymphocytes	no./l	$0\text{–}25 \times 10^6$	$0\text{–}20 \times 10^6$	$0\text{–}5 \times 10^6$	$0\text{–}5 \times 10^6$	$0\text{–}5 \times 10^6$
	(no./mm³)	(0–25)	(0–20)	(0–5)	(0–5)	(0–5)
Erythrocytes	no./l	$0\text{–}1000 \times 10^6$	$0\text{–}800 \times 10^6$	$0\text{–}5 \times 10^6$	$0\text{–}5 \times 10^6$	$0\text{–}5 \times 10^6$
	(no./mm³)	(0–1000)	(0–800)	(0–5)	(0–5)	(0–5)
Protein	mg/l	400–3000	450–1000	100–200	150–300	100–450
	(mg/dl)	(40–300)	(45–100)	(10–20)	(15–30)	(10–45)
Glucose	mmol/l		1.7–4.4	3.5–4.4	2.2–3.9	2.8–4.0
	(mg/dl)		(30–80)	(60–80)	(40–70)	(50–72)
IgG	mg/l			8–64	8–64	5–45
	(mg/dl)			(0.8–6.4)	(0.8–6.4)	(0.5–4.5)
IgG : total protein ratio						<15%

Normal CSF contains 0–5 mm³ erythrocytes, but a value of up to 50 is often found without any abnormal values in other CSF constituents

CSF glucose level is abnormal whenever less than 50% of blood glucose level

THERAPEUTIC DRUG MONITORING

Drug	Therapeutic range	Half-life	Sampling time	Time to steady state
Carbamazepine	15–50 μmol/l	12 hrs	Pre-dose	2–4 wks
Phenobarbitone	65–170 μmol/l	96 hrs	Pre-dose	3–4 wks
Phenytoin	40–80 μmol/l	7–42 hrs	Pre-dose	7–10 days
Lamotrigine	8–20 μmol/l		Pre-dose	
Valproic acid	350–700 μmol/l	8–20 hrs	Pre-dose	1–3 days
Cyclosporin A	180–350 μg/l*	2–6 hrs	Pre-dose	2–3 days
Digoxin	1.0–2.5 nmol/l / 0.8–2.0 μg/l	38 hrs	At least 6 hrs post-dose	8 days
L-DOPA	1.5–8.0 μmol/l	1–3 hrs	Timed — up to 3 hrs post-dose	
Lithium	0.3–1.6 mg/l / 0.5–1.2 mmol/l	18–36 hrs	Pre-dose	3–10 days
Theophylline	55–110 μmol/l	Variable	Pre-dose	2 days

*CyA HPLC– equivalent result applies to monotherapy in renal transplant patients only.
NB Toxic effects for some drugs may be observed at the upper limit of therapeutic levels.

BONE MARROW (NORMAL ADULT MYELOGRAM)

Total cell count	20 000–100 000 per mm³
Myelo-erythroid ratio	3:1–5:1

Differential count

Myeloid series (70%)		
Myeloblasts	0–2.5	
Promyelocytes	0.5–5.0	
Myelocytes		Granulocytes 57.4%
Neutrophil	2–8	
Eosinophil	0–1	
Metamyelocytes		
Neutrophil	10–25	
Eosinophil	0–2.5	
Polymorphonuclear		
Neutrophil	10–40	
Eosinophil	0–4	
Basophil	0–1	
Lymphocytes	5–20	Others 12.6%
Monocytes	0–5	
Plasma cells	0–1	
Erythroid series (19.1%)		
Haemocytoblasts	0–1	Nucleated red cells
Proerythroblasts	0–4	
Early and intermediate normoblasts	4–15	
Late normoblasts	7–19	
Not identifiable (10.9%)		

PROTHROMBIN TIME

British ratio (INR)	Clinical state
2.0–2.5	Prophylaxis of deep vein thrombosis including high risk surgery (e.g. for fractured femur)
2.0–3.0	Treatment of deep vein thrombosis, pulmonary embolism, transient ischaemic attacks
3.0–4.5	Recurrent deep vein thrombosis and pulmonary embolism; arterial disease including myocardial infarction; arterial grafts; cardiac prosthetic valves and grafts

*British ratios and international normalized ratios (INR) are virtually identical within the therapeutic range.

Proposed therapeutic ranges for prothrombin time (British Society for Haematology guidelines on oral anticoagulants, 1984).

GLUCOSE TOLERANCE TEST

	Capillary glucose (mmol/l)	Venous glucose (mmol/l)
Diabetes mellitus		
Fasting	>8.0	>8.0
2 hrs after glucose	>12.2	>11.0
Impaired glucose tolerance		
Fasting	<8.0	<8.0
2 hrs after glucose	8.9–12.2	8.0–11.0

BASAL METABOLIC RATE

Normal range	80–120%
Protein bound iodine	3–6 µg/100 ml

GASTRIC AND DUODENAL FLUID NORMAL VALUES (ADULT)

	Value	SI units
Amylase	> 1.2	Units/total sample
Basal gastric fluid	0.8 ± 0.6	µmol/s
Maximum gastric fluid	6.4 ± 1.4	µmol/s
pH duodenal fluid	5.6–7.6	l
Trypsin	0.35–1.60	% normal
Viscosity	3 or less	minutes

PANCREATIC FUNCTION (ADULT)

	Lower limit of normal
PABA/^{14}C excretion index	0.76
Lundh test (mean tryptic activity)	25 IU/ml
Secretin-pancreozymin test	
Volume in 1 hour	149 ml
Peak bicarbonate concentration	57.5 mmol/l
Peak tryptic activity	30 IU/ml
Total bicarbonate output in 30 minutes after secretin	5.7 mmol
Total trypsin output in 30 minutes after pancreozymin	2195 IU

FAECES

	Adults	Children
Total fat content	25%	33% dried weight
Split to unsplit ratio	3.1	2.1

LIVER FUNCTION TESTS NORMAL VALUES

Test	Normal range	Abnormality	Causes of abnormality
Total serum bilirubin, bilirubin esters	5-17 µmol/l, < 6 µmol/l	Unconjugated bilirubin Increased	(total esters) increases with over-production (e.g. haemolysis) and with failure of uptake or conjugation. Bilirubin esters increase with parenchymal liver disease or extrahepatic obstruction
Urine bilirubin	Negative result	Negative or increased	Positive result: most other causes of jaundice (many kinds of liver disease); unconjugated hyperbilirubinaemia: negative result
Serum aspartate aminotransferase (AST)	5-40 IU/l (37°C)	Increased	Myocardial infarction, Many kinds of liver disease
Serum alanine aminotransferase (ALT)	5-40 IU/l	Increased	Myopathies, Liver disease
Serum alkaline phosphatase	30-110 IU/l; levels are higher in children and adolescents	Increased	Liver disease — especially with obstruction to bile flow, Bone disease — Paget's disease, osteomalacia, some patients with bone secondaries or hyperparathyroidism, Pregnancy
Serum 5'-nucleotidase	1-15 IU/l (37°C)	Increased	Liver disease — especially with biliary obstruction. Often used to confirm that high phosphatase is hepatic in origin (unnecessary if alkaline phosphatase isoenzyme can be characterized)
Serum γ-glutamyl transferase	Men 0-65 IU/l, Women 0-40 IU/l (37°C)	Increased	Liver disease — most kinds, Chronic alcohol excess, Acute pancreatitis, Diabetes mellitus, Myocardial infarction, Enzyme-inducing drugs
Serum albumin	35-50 g/l	Decreased	Extensive liver damage, Nephrotic syndrome, Gastrointestinal disease, Fluid retention (which may complicate liver disease)
Serum caeruloplasmin	270-370 mg/l	Decreased	Wilson's disease
Total urine copper	13-21 µmol/l	Decreased	Wilson's disease
24-hour urine copper	0-0.4 µmol/24 h	Increased	Wilson's disease
Prothrombin time (PT), partial thromboplastin time (PTT)	PT: 10-14 s, PTT: 32-42 s	Increased	Liver disease, Vitamin K deficiency — corrected by 3 days of treatment unless synthesis is impaired due to hepatocyte damage. Hereditary disorders of the clotting mechanism

Ranges may vary from one laboratory to another.

GERIATRICS (NORMAL VALUES)

	Men		Women		Units
	Age 65–74	Age 75+	Age 65–74	Age 75+	
Albumin	36.3–44.5	36.0–47.4	37.4–45.8	37.6–45.4	g/l
Bicarbonate	22.5–28.1	23.1–28.3	22.3–28.3	22.3–27.3	mmol/l
Calcium	2.25–2.47	2.22–2.4	2.27–2.5	2.22–2.49	mmol/l
Cholesterol	4.26–9.19	4.08–8.47	4.7–11.47	4.6–11.0	mmol/l, 95% range
Chloride	99.1–105.1	99.9–105.5	99.5–105.3	99.5–105.5	mmol/l
Creatinine	58.3–160.0	68.9–162.6	38.0–83.9	38.8–139.6	mmol/l
Folate	2.5–21	Lower in elderly	2.5–21	Lower in elderly	mg/l
Haemoglobin	12.5–15.4	12.5–15.4	12.0–13.9	12.0–13.9	g/100 ml
Iron	8.7–30.1	8.7–30.1	Marginally lower in women until 60		µmol/l
Potassium	4.1–4.9	4.2–4.8	4.0–4.8	3.9–4.7	mmol/l
Phosphate	0.8–1.13	0.82–1.12	0.92–1.29	0.88–1.29	mmol/l
Prostatic specific antigen	0–4.5	0–6.5	—	—	ng/ml
Protein (total)	66.4–76.2	64.8–76.6	66.6–76.0	65.8–75.4	g/l
Sodium	137.4–143.6	138.3–143.3	138.4–143.6	137.9–143.9	mmol/l
Total iron-binding capacity	45–76	Falls with age	45–76	Falls with age	µmol/l
T4 Leads	2.9–7.0	2.9–7.0	2.9–7.0	2.9–7.0	mg/dl
T3 Uptake	92–117	92–117	92–117	92–117	
Urate	250–393	261–396.8	213–357	204.6–398.6	µmol/l
Urea	4.16–10.0	4.5–11.2	3.6–10.0	3.6–10.0	mmol/l, 95% range
Vitamin B12	200 ± 85	Progressive fall	166 ± 79	Progressive fall	ng/l

By courtesy of F. L. Willington, MD, Consultant Physician in Clinical Gerontology.

URINE ANALYSIS

Analyte	Range	Units	Results	Comments	Preservative
Albumin (micro)	<15	mg/l	<24 h	Random specimen	N
Albumin/creatinine ratio	<3.5	mg/mmol	<24 h	Assuming normal renal function	N
Aluminium	<1.0	µmol/l	As required	Contact lab.	S
Aluminium (water)	<1.0	µmol/l	As required	Contact lab.	S
Amino acids			As required	Contact lab.	H
Aminolaevulinic acid (ALA)	<40	µmol/24 h	<14 days	24 hour urine, protect from light	N
Amphetamines	Not detected		<72 h	Fresh specimen. Part of DoA Screen	N
Amylase	80–575	U/24 hrs	<24 h		H
Balance studies			As required	Contact lab for information	N
Barbiturates (screen)	Not detected		<72 h	Fresh specimen	N
Bence Jones protein	Not detected		As required	Early morning specimen Send serum and urine together	N
Benzodiazepines	Not detected		<72 h	Fresh specimen. Part of DoA Screen	N
Bilirubin	Not detected		On arrival	Fresh specimen	N
Bone studies			As required	Contact lab.	N
C-Amp (nephrogenous)	26–66(8–30)	nmol/GF	As required	Send blood and timed 2 h urine together	H
Cadmium	<0.15	pmol/24 hrs	As required	Contact ext 4240	S
Calcium	2.5–7.5	mmol/24 hrs	<24 h	On normal calcium intake	H
Calcium/creatinine ratio	0.3–0.7	mmol/mmol	<24 h	Assuming normal renal function	H
Calculus/stone analysis			As required	Contact lab for information	N
Cannabinoids	Not detected		<72 h	Fresh specimen. Part of DoA Screen	N
Catecholamines			14 days	Sulphuric acid preservative	S
Noradrenaline	120–590	nmol/24 hrs			
Adrenaline	30–190	nmol/24 hrs			
Dopamine	650–3270	nmol/24 hrs			
Citrate	1.0–5.0	mmol/24 hrs	As required	Transport to lab immediately	H
Cocaine metabolites	Not detected		<72 h	Fresh specimen. Part of DoA Screen	N
Copper	<1.0	µmol/l	As required		N
Corproporphyrin	<246	nmol/24 hrs	As required		N
Cortisol	<350	nmol/24 hrs	<7 days		H
Cortisol/creatinine ratio	<25	nmol/mmol	<7 days	Assuming normal renal function	H
Creatinine	9–18	mmol/24 hrs	<24 h	Proportional to body size	H
Cystine	<250	µmol/24 hrs	As required		H
Deoxypyridinoline/creatinine ratio	0.4–6.4	nmol/mmol	As required	2 h fasting, 2nd pass morning specimen Discard overnight urine	N
Drugs of abuse screen (DoA Screen)			<72 h	Fresh specimen — supervised. GCMS confirmation available	N
Glucose	Not detected		<24 h	Random specimen	N
Haemoglobin	Not detected		<24 h	Random specimen	N
Homocystine	Not detected		As required	Contact lab.	H

URINE ANALYSIS (cont'd)

Analyte	Range	Units	Results	Comments	Preservative
Homogentisic acid	Not detected		On arrival	Fresh specimen. Transport to lab immediately	H
Hydroxy indole acetic acid (5-HIAA)	<50	µmol/24 hrs	<7 days	Sulphuric acid preservative	S
Hydroxyproline	115–270	µmol/24 hrs	<14 days	Dietary restriction essential	H
Hydroxyproline/ creatinine ratio	<40	µmol/mmol	<14 days	Assuming normal renal function	H
Indican	Not detected		On arrival	Fresh specimen Transport to lab immediately	N
Iron	<0.5	µmol/24 hrs	As required	Contact lab.	S
Ketones	Not detected		On arrival	Random specimen	N
Laxative abuse	Not detected		As required	Fresh specimen	N
Lead	<0.54	µmol/l	As required	Contact lab.	S
Magnesium	3.0–5.0	mmol/24 hrs	As required		H
Manganese	<182	nmol/l	As required	Contact lab.	S
Mercury	<32	nmol/24 hrs	As required	Contact lab.	S
Methadone	Not detected		<72 h	Fresh specimen. Part of DoA Screen	N
Myoglobin	Not detected		On arrival	Random specimen	N
Nitrogen	10–15	g/24 hrs	As required	Varies with dietary intake	N
Nutritional assessment			As required	Contact lab.	H
Opiates	Not detected			Fresh specimen. Part of DoA Screen	N
Osmolality	250–750	mosmol/kg H_2O	<24 h		N
Oxalate	<500	µmol/24 hrs	<14 days	If elevated, associated with increased incidence of stone formation	H
Pancreolauryl test	Normal	≥30	As required	Contact bleep 117 for information	N
(T/k ratio)	Pancreatic insuff	<20			
Paraquat screen	Not detected		On arrival	Random specimen	N
Phaeochromocytoma screen			<14 days	Sulphuric acid preservative Contact lab.	S
Phenolphthalein	Not detected		<24 h	Random specimen	N
Phosphate		mmol/24 hrs	<24 h	Varies with dietary intake	H
Porphobilinogen	<16	µmol/24 hrs	<14 days	24 hr urine, protect from light	N
Porphyrin (screen)	Not detected		<24 h	Fresh specimen, protect from light	N
Potassium	25–100	mmol/24 hrs	<24 h		H
Pregnancy test	Positive/ negative		<24 h	Early morning urine specimen	N
Protein	<0.15	g/24 hrs	<24 h		H
Pyridinoline/ creatinine ratio	5.0–21.8	nmol/mmol	As required	2 hr fasting, 2nd pass morning specimen Discard overnight urine	N
Pyrophosphate	<130	µmol/24 hrs	As required		H
Reducing substances	Not detected		<24 h	Random specimen	N
Renal stone profile			As required	Contact lab.	H
Selenium	<1.3	µmol/l	As required	Varies with dietary intake, contact lab.	N
Silicon	100–700	µmol/24 hrs	As required	Varies with dietary intake, contact lab.	N

URINE ANALYSIS (cont'd)

Analyte	Range	Units	Results	Comments	Preservative
Sodium	130–220	mmol/24 hrs	<24 h		H
Toxic elements			As required	Contact lab.	S
Trace elements			As required	Contact lab.	S
U & E		<24 hrs		Contact lab.	H
Urea	250–500	mmol/24 hrs	<24 h	Varies with dietary intake	H
Uric acid		mmol/24 hrs	<24 h	Varies with dietary intake	H
Urobilinogen	Not detected		<24 h	Fresh specimen	N
Xylose	>8	mmol/5 hrs	As required	5 hour urine collection, following a 5 g dose	N

H, Hibitane; S, special preservative; and N, no preservative.

NORMAL VALUES IN RENAL MEDICINE

		Range	Units
Plasma			
Sodium*		135–145	mmol/l
Potassium*		3.5–5.0	mmol/l
Chloride*		96–106	mmol/l
Bicarbonate*		23–29	mmol/l
Ammonium†	Men	34–58	µmol/l
	Women	17–51	µmol/l
Urea‡		2.5–7.0	mmol/l
		2.9–8.9	mmol/l
		2.0–4.2	mmol/l
Creatinine†		60–130	µmol/l
		18–64	µmol/l
Urate‡	Men	0.15–0.42	mmol/l
	Women	0.12–0.39	mmol/l
Base‡		145–148	mmol/l
Osmolality*		280–295	mOsmol/kg
Serum			
Total calcium*		2.12–2.61	mmol/l
Ionized calcium*		1.14–1.30	mmol/l
Inorganic phosphate†		0.8–1.4	mmol/l
Total protein*		60–80	g/l
Albumin*		35–50	g/l
Globulin*		20–40	g/l
IgG†		9.5–16.5	g/l
IgA†		0.9–4.5	g/l
IgM		0.6–2.0	g/l
Sulphate		50–150	µmol/l
C3		0.94–2.14	g/l
C4*		0.16–0.5	g/l
Aluminium‡		0.07–0.55	µmol/l

NORMAL VALUES IN RENAL MEDICINE (cont'd)

	Range	Units
24-hour urinary excretion		
Protein*	Up to 200	mg
Albumin*	Up to 25	mg
Calcium‡	2.5–7.5	mmol
Oxalate‡	0.22–0.44	mmol
Cystine†	0.04–0.42	mmol
Glomerular filtration rate and other renal function tests		
GFR† Men Age 20	117–170	ml/min/1.73 m²
Age 50	96–138	ml/min/1.73 m²
Age 70	70–110	ml/min/1.73 m²
Women Age 20	104–158	ml/min/1.73 m²
Age 50	90–130	ml/min/1.73 m²
Age 70	74–114	ml/min/1.73 m²
Pregnant	About 20% higher	
Maximum urine concentration†	>800	mOsmol/kg
Minimum urine pH‡	<5.3	

*Variables which are little affected by age, sex, diet and size; published normal ranges can be used and some should be memorized.
†Variables which vary with sex, age or size; the more important and better established ones are shown subdivided or corrected for size.
‡Variables that depend on diet; for these your local hospital reference range is usually a better guide than any culled from published data.

NORMAL ECG

Electrocardiograph

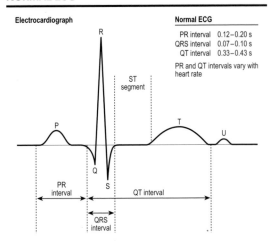

Normal ECG

PR interval	0.12–0.20 s
QRS interval	0.07–0.10 s
QT interval	0.33–0.43 s

PR and QT intervals vary with heart rate

CONVENTIONAL CONNECTIONS IN ELECTROCARDIOGRAPHY

Lead I	Right arm to left arm
Lead II	Right arm to left arm
Lead III	Left arm to left leg
AVR	Right arm to left arm and left leg together
AVL	Left arm to right arm and left leg together
AVF	Left leg to right arm and left arm
V_1	4th right intercostal space parasternally to I, II and III
V_2	4th left intercostal space parasternally to I, II and III
V_3	Halfway between V_2 and the 5th space midclavicular line to I, II and III
V_4	5th left interspace midclavicular line to I, II and III
V_5	Anterior axillary line at the same horizontal plane as V_4 to I, II and III
V_6	Mid-axillary line in the same plane to I, II and III
V_7	Posterior axillary line in the same plane to I, II and III

CALCULATION OF HEART RATE

R–R interval (s)*	Number of 'big'† squares	Heart rate (beats per minute)
0.2	1	300
0.4	2	150
0.6	3	100
0.8	4	75
1.0	5	60
1.2	6	50
1.4	7	43
1.6	8	37

*Check standard paper speed 25 mm/s.
†Count the number of 'big' squares between each R wave.

ANALYSIS OF THE NORMAL ECG

Identify rhythm	Sinus rhythm
	  P wave rate constant
	  P wave precedes each QRS complex
	  Single P wave to each QRS complex
	Heart rate 60–100 per minute

Assess P wave	<0.12 s duration <2.5 mm height in lead II
Measure PR interval	0.12–20 s
Assess QRS complexes	Duration <0.12 s S wave >R wave lead V_1 R wave V_5, V_6 <25 mm Q waves <0.04 s duration <25% height ensuing R wave
Calculate QRS axis	¯30°–¯90°
Check QT interval	0.38–0.42 s
Assess ST segments	Deviation <0.1 mm from isoelectric line
Assess T waves	Upright V_3–V_6, I, II, aVF — generally with QRS vector

PRINCIPAL ECG MANIFESTATIONS OF MYOCARDIAL INFARCTION (MI)

	Morphology	Evolution
ST segment	Elevation leads facing infarct zone Slight curvature, convex upwards Reciprocal ST depression leads opposing infarct zone ST depression may be principal change in non-Q wave MI	Usually first ECG manifestation Usually lasts a few days only Prolonged ST elevation may indicate extensive MI, presence LV aneurysm
T waves	Wide range of changes seen Tall, peaked in early MI Deep symmetrical T inversion often seen adjacent to infarct zone	Widespread T inversion first appears after the first 24 h Changes may persist for many weeks
Q waves; loss of R wave voltage	Pathological Q >0.04 s, amplitude >25% subsequent R wave height	Follow ST elevation Changes are usually persistent but may disapper with infarct scar contraction

CARDIAC CATHETERIZATION/NORMAL VALUES OF PRESSURES AND SATURATIONS

Location	Pressure (mmHg)	Saturation
Inferior vena cava		
Superior vena cava		
Right atrium		
a	2–10	
v	2–10	
Mean	0–8	
Right ventricle		74
Systolic	15–30	
End diastolic	0–8	
Pulmonary artery		
Systolic	15–30	
End diastolic	3–12	
Mean	9–16	
Pulmonary capillary wedge		
a	3–15	
v	3–12	
Mean	1–10	
Left ventricle		98
Systolic	100–140	
End diastolic	3–12	
Aorta		
Systolic	100–140	
End diastolic	60–90	

CARDIAC CATHETERIZATION: GRADIENTS (mmHg) ACROSS STENOTIC VALVES

Valve	Normal gradient	Stenotic gradient		
		Mild	Moderate	Severe
Aortic	0	<30	30–70	>70
Mitral	0	<5	5–15	>15
Prosthetic	5–10			

Intracardiac electrophysiological studies of the type and origin arrhythmias and aberrant pathways can be performed at catheterization

RECOMMENDATIONS RELATING TO CARDIAC DISORDERS WHICH MAY PREVENT THE HOLDING OF AN ORDINARY DRIVING LICENCE

There is a requirement that patients with the following cardiac disorders should not drive a motor vehicle and should notify their disorder to the Driver and Vehicle Licensing Centre (DVLA)

1 Within one month of a heart attack, pacemaker insertion, heart surgery or angioplasty
2 When angina is easily provoked during driving and emotion
3 When drugs for any cardiac disorder causes symptoms
4 When there have been one or more episodes of unexplained syncope
5 When heart block exists or an implantable cardioverter defibrillator has been implanted

PULSE (NORMAL RATE PER MINUTE)

Age	Rate per minute
Birth	140-130
1 month	130-120
1 year	120-110
2 years	108-90
3 years	90-80
7 years	80-80
7-20 years	85-80
21-60 years	85-80
over 60 years	70-80
	66-60

BLOOD PRESSURE (NORMAL RANGE OF ARTERIAL PRESSURE)

Age (years)	Men		Women	
	Systolic	Diastolic	Systolic	Diastolic
16-19	105-135	60-85	100-130	60-85
20-24	110-140	60-90	102-130	60-85
25-29	108-140	60-90	102-130	60-98
30-34	110-145	60-90	102-135	60-98
35-39	110-145	68-89	105-140	65-90
40-44	110-150	76-94	105-150	65-96
45-49	110-155	76-96	105-155	65-96
50-54	115-160	70-98	110-165	70-100
55-59	115-165	70-98	110-170	70-100
60-65	115-170	70-100	115-175	70-100

BLOOD PRESSURE FOLLOW UP

Measurement	Range (mmHg)	Recommended follow up*
	Diastolic blood pressure (DBP)	
	<85	Recheck within two years
	85-89	Recheck within one year
	90-104	Confirm promptly (not to exceed two months)
	105-114	Evaluate or refer promptly to source of care (not to exceed two weeks)
	<115	Evaluate or refer immediately to source of care
Second time	Systolic blood pressure (SBP) when DBP is <90	
	<140	Recheck within two years
	140-199	Confirm promptly (not to exceed two months)
	>200	Evaluate or refer promptly to source of care (not to exceed two weeks)
	Diastolic blood pressure	
	<85	Recheck within two years†
	85-89	Recheck within one year
	>90	Evaluate or refer promptly to a source of care
First time	Systolic blood pressure within DBP is <90	
Measurement	<140	Recheck within one year
	>140	Evaluate or refer promptly to source of care

*If recommended follow up for DBP and SBPs are different, the shorter recommended time period takes precedence and referral supersedes a recheck recommendation.

†Rechecking within one year is recommended for patients at increased risk of progressing to higher blood pressure levels, including family history of hypertension or cardiovascular event, weight gain or obesity, black race, use of an oral contraceptive and excessive ethanol consumption.

The prevention of coronary heart disease. The Royal College of General Practitioners, 1988. (with permission.)

BLOOD GASES

	Arterial		Mixed venous	
	Pressure (kPa)	Content (mmol/l)	Pressure (kPa)	Content (mmol/l)
O_2	11.9–13.2	8.9–9.4	5.0–5.6	6.7–7.2
CO_2	4.8–6.3	21.6–22.5	5.6–6.7	23.3–24.2
pH	—	7.35–7.45	—	7.34–7.42
H^+ nmol/l	—	36–44	—	38–46
HCO_3^- mmol/l	—	24–30	—	24–30

RESPIRED GASES

	Pressures (kPa)			Percentages		
	Air	Alveolar	Mixed expired	Air	Alveolar	Mixed expired
O_2	19.9	13–15	15–16	20.93	13–15	16–17
N_2	75.0	78–9	77	79.04	78–9	80
CO_2	—	4–6	2.8–3.7	0.03	4–6	3–4
H_2O	—	6.3	6.3	—	6.3	6.3

GAS EXCHANGE

Measurement	Notation	Mean value/ range	Units	Comments
Respiratory frequency	fR	12–20	/min	
Minute volume	$\dot{V}_E$	6–10	l/min	↑ With exercise, fever, size
Tidal volume	V_T	0.35–0.65	l	
Alveolar minute volume	$\dot{V}_A$	4–7	l/min	
Anatomical dead space	V_D	2	ml/kg	
Volume dead space gas/tidal volume	V_D/V_T	0.3		
O_2 consumption	$\dot{n}O_2$	11–13	mmol/min	
CO_2 production	$\dot{n}O_2$	9–11 (88–110 ml/m²)	mmol/min	↑ With fever, exercise
Alveolar–arterial O_2 difference	$A\text{-}a\,DO_2$	(1) 0.7–2.0 (2) 1.3–8.8	kPa kPa	Breathing air Breathing O_2
Physiological R → L shunt	$\dot{Q}_s/\dot{Q}_t$	1–2%		
Respiratory quotient	$\dfrac{\dot{n}CO_2:R}{\dot{n}O_2}$	0.8		Range 0.7–1.0

RESPIRATION (NORMAL RATE PER MINUTE)

Age	Rate per minute
Birth	50–40
1–12 months	35–25
1–4 years	25
5–15 years	25–20
Adult	18

RESPIRATORY MEDICINE 33

LUNG FUNCTION: CHILDREN

| Boys and girls aged 2–15 years | | | Boys aged 7–15 years | | Girls aged 7–15 years | |
| Height | | PEFR Litres/min | | | | |
m	ft/in		FEV_1	FVC	FEV_1	FVC
0.90	2'11"	92				
0.95	3'1"	107				
1.00	3'3"	124				
1.05	3'5"	146				
1.10	3'7"	169	1.06	1.30	1.02	1.21
1.15	3'9"	192	1.20	1.47	1.15	1.36
1.20	3'11"	215	1.35	1.65	1.30	1.52
1.25	4'1"	238	1.51	1.84	1.45	1.69
1.30	4'3"	260	1.68	2.05	1.61	1.88
1.35	4'5"	283	1.86	2.27	1.79	2.07
1.40	4'7"	306	2.06	2.51	1.97	2.28
1.45	4'9"	329	2.27	2.76	2.17	2.49
1.50	4'11"	352	2.50	3.02	2.38	2.73
1.55	5'1"	374	2.73	3.31	2.61	2.97
1.60	5'3"	397	2.99	3.61	2.84	3.23
1.65	5'5"	419	3.25	3.92	3.09	3.50
1.70	5'7"	442	3.53	4.25	3.35	3.78
1.75	5'9"	465	3.83	4.60	3.63	4.08
1.80	5'11"	488	4.14	4.97	3.92	4.39

PEFR, Peak expiratory flow-rate; FEV_1, forced expiratory volume in one second; and FVC, forced vital capacity.

LUNG FUNCTION IN ADULTS

	Men	Women
Forced expiratory volume in one second (FEV_1)	3.5±1.5 l	2.5±1.0 l
Forced vital capacity (FVC)	4.5±1.5 l	3.5±1.0 l
Forced expiratory flow (FEF)	4.3±0.51 l/sec	3.48±0.47 l/sec
Peak expiratory flow-rate (PEFR)	550±150 l/min	400±100 l/min

CHARACTERISTIC CHANGES IN TYPICAL PULMONARY DISORDERS

Disorder	Vital capacity*	Forced expiratory volume†	Maximum voluntary ventilation*	Residual volume*	CO diffusing capacity‡	Arterial pO_2 (mmHg)	Arterial pCO_2 (mmHg)
Normal	>80	>75	>80	80–120	25–30	80–100	38–42
Restrictive disorders							
Mild	60–80	>75	>80	80–120	↓E	80–100	38–42
Moderate	50–60	>75	>80	70–80	↓R	↓	↓
Severe	35–50	>75	60–80	60–70	↓	↓	↓
Very severe	<35	>75	<60	<60	↓↓	↓↓	↑
Obstructive disorders							
Mild	>80	60–75	65–80	120–150	25–30	↓E	38–42
Moderate	>80	40–60	45–65	150–175	25–30	↓	↓
Severe	↓	<40	30–45	>200	↓	↓	↑E
Very severe	↓	<40	<30	>200	↓	↓↓	↑R

E = Exercise, R = Rest.
* % Predicted.
† % Vital capacity.
‡ ml/min/mmHg Mean value (breath held 10 s).

MALE PREDICTED NORMAL VALUES

Age Height (cm)	150	155	160	165	170	175	180	185	190	195
18–25 FVC	3.65	3.94	4.23	4.51	4.80	5.09	5.38	5.67	5.95	6.24
25 FEV1	3.24	3.45	3.67	3.88	4.10	4.31	4.53	4.74	4.96	5.17
25 FEF 25–75%	4.54	4.63	4.73	4.83	4.92	5.02	5.12	5.21	5.31	5.41
25 PEF	479	498	516	534	553	571	590	608	626	645
26–29 FVC	3.55	3.83	4.12	4.41	4.70	4.99	5.27	5.56	5.85	6.14
29 FEV1	3.12	3.33	3.55	3.76	3.98	4.19	4.41	4.62	4.84	5.05
29 FEF 25–75%	4.36	4.46	4.56	4.65	4.75	4.85	4.95	5.04	5.14	5.24
29 PEF	469	487	506	524	542	561	579	598	616	635
29–33 FVC	3.44	3.73	4.02	4.31	4.59	4.88	5.17	5.46	5.75	6.03
33 FEV1	3.00	3.22	3.43	3.65	3.86	4.08	4.29	4.51	4.72	4.94
33 FEF 25–75%	4.19	4.29	4.39	4.48	4.58	4.68	4.77	4.87	4.97	5.06
33 PEF	458	477	495	514	532	551	569	587	606	624
34–37 FVC	3.34	3.63	3.91	4.20	4.49	4.78	5.07	5.35	5.64	5.93
37 FEV1	2.89	3.10	3.32	3.53	3.75	3.96	4.18	4.39	4.61	4.82
37 FEF 25–75%	4.02	4.12	4.21	4.31	4.41	4.50	4.60	4.70	4.80	4.89
37 PEF	448	467	485	503	522	540	559	577	596	614
38–41 FVC	3.23	3.52	3.81	4.10	4.39	4.67	4.96	5.25	5.54	5.83
41 REV1	2.77	2.99	3.20	3.42	3.63	3.85	4.06	4.28	4.49	4.71
41 FEF 25–75%	3.85	3.94	4.04	4.14	4.24	4.33	4.43	4.53	4.62	4.72
41 PEF	438	456	475	493	512	530	548	567	585	604
42–45 FVC	3.13	3.42	3.71	3.99	4.28	4.57	4.86	5.15	5.43	5.72
45 FEV1	2.66	2.87	3.09	3.30	3.52	3.73	3.95	4.16	4.38	4.59
45 FEF 25–75%	3.68	3.77	3.87	3.97	4.06	4.16	4.26	4.35	4.45	4.55
45 PEF	428	446	464	483	501	520	538	556	575	593
46–49 FVC	3.03	3.31	3.60	3.89	4.18	4.47	4.75	5.04	5.33	5.62
49 FEV1	2.54	2.75	2.97	3.18	3.40	3.61	3.83	4.04	4.26	4.47
49 FEF 25–75%	3.50	3.60	3.70	3.79	3.89	3.99	4.09	4.18	4.28	4.38
49 PEF	417	436	454	472	491	509	528	546	565	583
50–53 FVC	2.92	3.21	3.50	3.79	4.07	4.36	4.65	4.94	5.23	5.51
53 FEV1	2.42	2.64	2.85	3.07	3.28	3.50	3.71	3.93	4.14	4.36
53 FEF 25–75%	3.33	3.43	3.53	3.62	3.72	3.82	3.91	4.01	4.11	4.20
53 PEF	407	425	444	462	481	499	517	536	554	573
54–57 FVC	2.82	3.11	3.39	3.68	3.97	4.26	4.55	4.83	5.12	5.41
57 FEV1	2.31	2.52	2.74	2.95	3.17	3.38	3.60	3.81	4.03	4.24
57 FEF 25–75%	3.16	3.26	3.35	3.45	3.55	3.64	3.74	3.84	3.94	4.03
57 PEF	397	415	433	452	470	489	507	525	544	562
58–61 FVC	2.71	3.00	3.29	3.58	3.87	4.15	4.44	4.73	5.02	5.31
61 FEV1	2.19	2.41	2.62	2.84	3.05	3.27	3.48	3.70	3.91	4.13
61 FEF 25–75%	2.99	3.08	3.18	3.28	3.38	3.47	3.57	3.67	3.76	3.86
61 PEF	386	405	423	441	460	478	497	515	534	552
62–65 FVC	2.61	2.90	3.19	3.47	3.76	4.05	4.34	4.63	4.91	5.20
65 FEV1	2.08	2.29	2.51	2.72	2.94	3.15	3.37	3.58	3.80	4.01
65 FEF 25–75%	2.82	2.91	3.01	3.11	3.20	3.30	3.40	3.49	3.59	3.69
65 PEF	376	394	413	431	450	468	486	505	523	542
66–69 FVC	2.51	2.79	3.08	3.37	3.66	3.95	4.23	4.52	4.81	5.10
69 FEV1	1.96	2.17	2.39	2.60	2.82	3.03	3.25	3.46	3.68	3.89
69 FEF 25–75%	2.64	2.74	2.84	2.93	3.03	3.13	3.23	3.32	3.42	3.52
69 PEF	366	384	402	421	439	458	476	495	513	531

FVC, Forced vital capacity; FEV_1 forced expiratory volume in one second
PEFR peak expiratory flow rate in litres per minute

The European Respiratory Journal (1993) Vol 6 Sup 16 Standardized Lung Function Testing. Official Statement of the European Respiratory Society

FEMALE PREDICTED NORMAL VALUES

Age Height (cm)	150	155	160	165	170	175	180	185	190	195
18–25 FVC	3.11	3.33	3.55	3.77	3.99	4.21	4.43	4.66	4.88	5.10
25 FEV1	2.70	2.90	3.10	3.29	3.49	3.69	3.89	4.08	4.28	4.48
25 FEF 25–75%	3.95	4.01	4.07	4.13	4.20	4.26	4.32	4.38	4.45	4.51
25 PEF	383	400	416	433	449	466	482	499	515	532
26–29 FVC	3.00	3.22	3.44	3.67	3.89	4.11	4.33	4.55	4.77	4.99
29 FEV1	2.60	2.80	3.00	3.19	3.39	3.59	3.79	3.98	4.18	4.38
29 FEF 25–75%	3.81	3.87	3.93	4.00	4.06	4.12	4.18	4.25	4.31	4.37
29 PEF	376	393	409	426	442	459	475	492	508	525
29–33 FVC	2.90	3.12	3.34	3.56	3.78	4.00	4.23	4.45	4.67	4.89
33 FEV1	2.50	2.70	2.90	3.09	3.29	3.49	3.69	3.88	4.08	4.28
33 FEF 25–75%	3.67	3.74	3.80	3.86	3.92	3.99	4.05	4.11	4.17	4.24
33 PEF	369	386	402	419	435	452	468	485	501	518
34–37 FVC	2.79	3.01	3.24	3.46	3.68	3.90	4.12	4.34	4.57	4.79
37 FEV1	2.40	2.60	2.80	2.99	3.19	3.39	3.59	3.78	3.98	4.18
37 FEF 25–75%	3.54	3.60	3.66	3.72	3.79	3.85	3.91	3.97	4.04	4.10
37 PEF	362	378	395	411	428	444	461	477	494	510
38–41 FVC	2.69	2.91	3.13	3.35	3.58	3.80	4.02	4.24	4.46	4.68
41 REV1	2.30	2.50	2.70	2.89	3.09	3.29	3.49	3.68	3.88	4.08
41 FEF 25–75%	3.40	3.46	3.53	3.59	3.65	3.71	3.78	3.84	3.90	3.96
41 PEF	355	371	388	404	421	437	454	470	487	503
42–45 FVC	2.59	2.81	3.03	3.25	3.47	3.69	3.91	4.14	4.36	4.58
45 FEV1	2.20	2.40	2.60	2.79	2.99	3.19	3.39	3.58	3.78	3.98
45 FEF 25–75%	3.27	3.33	3.39	3.45	3.52	3.58	3.64	3.70	3.77	3.83
45 PEF	347	364	380	397	413	430	446	463	479	496
46–49 FVC	2.48	2.70	2.92	3.15	3.37	3.59	3.81	4.03	4.25	4.47
49 FEV1	2.10	2.30	2.50	2.69	2.89	3.09	3.29	3.48	3.68	3.88
49 FEF 25–75%	3.13	3.19	3.25	3.32	3.38	3.44	3.50	3.57	3.63	3.69
49 PEF	340	357	373	390	406	423	439	456	472	489
50–53 FVC	2.38	2.60	2.82	3.04	3.26	3.48	3.71	3.93	4.15	4.37
53 FEV1	2.00	2.20	2.40	2.59	2.79	2.99	3.19	3.38	3.58	3.78
53 FEF 25–75%	2.99	3.06	3.12	3.18	3.24	3.31	3.37	3.43	3.49	3.56
53 PEF	333	350	366	383	399	416	432	449	465	482
54–57 FVC	2.27	2.49	2.72	2.94	3.16	3.38	3.60	3.82	4.05	4.27
57 FEV1	1.90	2.10	2.30	2.49	2.69	2.89	3.09	3.28	3.46	3.66
57 FEF 25–75%	2.86	2.92	2.98	3.04	3.11	3.17	3.23	3.29	3.36	3.42
57 PEF	326	342	359	375	392	408	425	441	458	474
58–61 FVC	2.17	2.39	2.61	2.83	3.06	3.28	3.50	3.72	3.94	4.16
61 FEV1	1.80	2.00	2.20	2.39	2.59	2.79	2.99	3.18	3.38	3.58
61 FEF 25–75%	2.72	2.78	2.85	2.91	2.97	3.03	3.10	3.16	3.22	3.28
61 PEF	319	335	352	368	385	401	418	434	451	467
62–65 FVC	2.07	2.29	2.51	2.73	2.95	3.17	3.39	3.62	3.84	4.06
65 FEV1	1.70	1.90	2.10	2.29	2.49	2.69	2.89	3.08	3.28	3.48
65 FEF 25–75%	2.59	2.65	2.71	2.77	2.84	2.90	2.96	3.02	3.09	3.15
65 PEF	311	328	344	361	377	394	410	427	443	460
66–69 FVC	1.96	2.18	2.40	2.63	2.85	3.07	3.29	3.51	3.73	3.95
69 FEV1	1.60	1.80	2.00	2.19	2.39	2.59	2.79	2.98	3.18	3.38
69 FEF 25–75%	2.45	2.51	2.57	2.64	2.70	2.76	2.82	2.89	2.95	3.01
69 PEF	304	321	337	354	370	387	403	420	436	453

FVC, Forced vital capacity; FEV_1 forced expiratory volume in one second
PEFR peak expiratory flow rate in litres per minute
The European Respiratory Journal (1993) Vol 6 Sup 16 Standardized
Lung Function Testing. Official Statement of the European Respiratory
Society

DERMATOMES

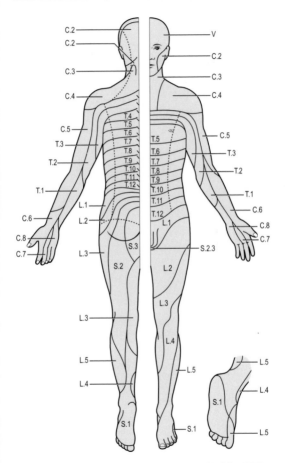

Adapted from Hope RA Oxford Handbook of Clinical Medicine (1989),
pp 410–411 (by permission of Oxford University Press)

TESTING PERIPHERAL NERVES

Nerve root	Muscle	Test — by asking the patient to:
C3,4	Trapezius	Shrug shoulder, adduct scapula
C4,5	Rhomboids	Brace shoulder back
C5,6,7	Serratus anterior	Push forward against resistance
C5,6,7,8	Pectoralis major (clavicular head)	Adduct arm from above horizontal and forward
C6,7,8 T1	Pectoralis major (sternocostal head)	Adduct arm below horizontal
C5,6	Supraspinatus	Abduct the arm the first 15°
C5,6	Infraspinatus	Externally rotate arm, elbow at side
C6,7,8	Latissimus dorsi	Adduct horizontal and lateral arm
C5,6	Biceps	Flex supinated forearm
C5,6	Deltoid	Abduct arm between 15° and 90°
Radial nerve		
C7,8	Triceps	Extend elbow against resistance
C5,6	Brachioradialis	Flex elbow with forearm halfway between pronation and supination
C6,7	Extensor carpi radialis longus	Extend wrist to radial side with fingers extended
C5	Supinator	Arm by side, resist hand pronation
C6,7,8	Extensor digitorum	Keep fingers extended at MCP joint
C7,8	Extensor carpi ulnaris	Extend wrist to ulnar side
C7,8	Abductor pollicis longus	Abduct thumb at 90° to palm
C7,8	Extensor pollicis brevis	Extend thumb at MCP joint
C7,8	Extensor pollicis longus	Resist thumb flexion at IP joint
Median nerve		
C6,7	Pronator teres	Keep arm pronated against resistance
C6,7,8	Flexor carpi radialis	Flex wrist towards radial side
C7,8 T1	Flexor digitorum sublimis	Resist extension at PIP joint (while you fix the proximal phalanx)
C8 T1	Flexor digitorum profundus I and II	Resist extension at the DIP joint
C8 T1	Flexor pollicis longus	Resist thumb extension at interphalangeal joint (fix proximal phalanx)
C8 T1	Abductor pollicis brevis	Abduct thumb (nail at 90° to palm)
C8 T1	Opponens pollicis	Thumb touches 5th fingertip (nail) parallel to palm
C8 T1	1st and 2nd lumbricals	Extend PIP joint against resistance with MCP joint held hyper-extended
Ulnar nerve		
C7,8	Flexor carpi ulnaris	Abducting little finger, see tendon when all fingers extended
C8 T1	Flexor digitorum profundus III and IV	Fix middle phalanx of little finger, resisting extension of distal phalanx
C8 T1	Dorsal interossei	Abduct fingers (use index finger)
C8 T1	Palmar interossei	Adduct fingers (use index finger)
C8 T1	Abductor digiti minimi	Abduct little finger
C8 T1	Opponens digiti minimi	With fingers extended, carry little finger in front of other fingers
L4,5 S1	Gluteus medius and minimus (superior gluteal nerve)	Internal rotation at hip, hip abduction
L5 S1,2	Gluteus maximus (inferior gluteal nerve)	Extension at hip (lie the prone)
L2,3,4	Adductors (obturator nerve)	Adduct leg against resistance
Femoral nerve		
L1,2,3	Ilio-psoas	Flex hip with knee flexed and lower leg supported (patient lies on back)
L2,3	Sartorius	Flex knee with hip external rotated
L2,3,4	Quadriceps femoris	Extend knee against resistance
Sciatic nerve		
L4,5 S1,2	Hamstrings	Flex knee against resistance
L4,5	Tibialis posterior	Invert plantar-flexed foot
L4,5	Tibialis anterior	Dorsiflex ankle

TESTING PERIPHERAL NERVES (cont'd)

Nerve root	Muscle	Test — by asking the patient to:
L5 S1	Extensor digitorum longus	Dorsiflex toes against resistance
L5 S1	Extensor hallucis longus	Dorsiflex hallux against resistance
L5 S1	Peroneus longus and brevis	Evert foot against resistance
S1	Extensor digitorum brevis	Dorsiflex hallux (muscle of foot)
S1,2	Gastrocnemius	Plantar flex ankle joint
S1,2	Flexor digitorum longus	Flex terminal joints of toes
S1,2	Small muscles of foot	Make sole of foot into a cup

Adapted from Hope RA Testing peripheral nerves. Oxford Handbook of Clinical Medicine (1989), pp 408–409 (by permission of Oxford University Press)

MOTOR FUNCTION: ROOT AND PERIPHERAL NERVE SUPPLY OF MUSCLE GROUPS

Movement	Muscle group	Root value*	Peripheral nerve†
Arms			
Shoulder abduction	Deltoid	C5	Axillary
Elbow flexion	Biceps	C5–6	—
	Brachioradialis		Radial
Shoulder adduction	Latissimus dorsi	C7	—
	Pectoralis		—
Elbow extension	Triceps	C7	Radial
Wrist extension	Extensor muscles of the forearm	C7	Radial
Wrist flexion	Flexor muscles of the forearm	C7 (8)	Median and ulnar
Finger extension	Extensor muscles of the forearm	C7 (8)	Radial
Finger flexion	Flexor muscles of the forearm	C8	Median and ulnar
Thumb abduction	Abductor pollicis brevis	T1	Median
Finger adduction	Interossei	T1	Median and ulnar
	Abductor digiti minimi		
Legs			
Hip flexion	Iliopsoas	L2 (3)	—
Hip adduction	Adductors	L2,3	Obturator
Knee extension	Quadriceps	L3,4	Femoral
Ankle inversion	Tibialis anterior	L4,5	Sciatic (peroneal)
	Tibialis posterior		Sciatic (tibial)
Ankle dorsiflexion	Tibialis anterior (and other anterior compartment muscles)	L4 (5)	Sciatic (peroneal)
Great toe dorsiflexion	Extensor hallucis longus	L5	Sciatic (peroneal)
Hip abduction	Glutei	L4,5	—
Hip extension	Glutei	L5, S1	—
Knee flexion	Hamstrings	S1 (L5)	Sciatic
Ankle eversion	Peroneus longus	L5, S1	Sciatic (peroneal)
Ankle plantarflexion	Gastrocnemius	S1,2	Sciatic (tibial)

* Roots with the most important contribution with subsidiary roots in parentheses.
† Clinically significant nerves only listed (main nerve listed with branches in parentheses).

ROOT AND PERIPHERAL NERVE SUPPLY OF TENDON JERKS

Tendon jerk	Root	Muscle group	Peripheral nerve
Biceps	C5,6	Biceps	Musculocutaneous
Triceps	C7	Triceps	Radial
Supinator	C5	Brachioradialis	Radial
Finger	C8	Long finger flexors	Median and ulnar
Knee	L4	Quadriceps	Femoral
Ankle	S1	Gastrocnemius	Sciatic (tibial branch)

NORMAL ADULT EEG

The main feature of the EEG of the alert adult is the presence of:

Symmetrical alpha rhythm, prominent posteriorly and attenuated by eye opening — in addition to this there may be:

- beta rhythm — usually in small quantities, of low amplitude and mainly frontal
- mu rhythm — usually sporadic and in small quantities
- lambda waves — usually in small numbers
- theta and delta rhythms — should be minimal or absent

On overbreathing, a symmetrical and high amplitude theta or delta activity may occur mainly in the frontal regions

During drowsiness and sleep, this pattern is altered. The following stages of sleep are recognised:

Stage 1	Low amplitude mixed frequency with alpha rhythm occupying less than 50% of the record
Stage 2	Low amplitude mixed frequency record with sleep spindles, K complexes
Stage 3	Between 20 and 50% of the record containing delta activity (of 2 Hz or less) with an amplitude greater than 75 µV and vertex sharp waves
Stage 4	Over 50% of the recording containing delta activity (of 2 Hz or less) with an amplitude greater than 75 µV

Definitions:

Alpha rhythm: rhythm with frequency of 8–13 cycles/s
Beta rhythm: rhythm with frequency of 14 cycles/s or more
Delta rhythm: rhythm with frequency of less than 4 cycles/s
K complex: a brief generalized complex of high voltage delta waves and sleep spindles
Lambda waves: positive triangular shaped waves seen in the posterior regions when the eyes are open and the subject is concentrating on visual material
Mu rhythm: a rhythm at 7–11 cycles/s in the Rolandic regions, usually persisting with eye opening and attenuated by movement of the contralateral limb
Sleep spindle: 12–14 cycles/s activity often asymmetrical and maximal frontally
Theta rhythm: frequency of 4–8 cycles/s
Vertex sharp waves: synchronous and symmetrical sharp waves phase reversing across the vertex

SERUM ANTICONVULSANT LEVELS: UPPER LIMIT OF OPTIMUM RANGE

Phenobarbitone	130 µmol/l
Primidone	60 µmol/l
Primidone (derived phenobarbitone)*	30 µmol/l
Phenytoin	570 µmol/l
Ethosuximide	60 µmol/l
Carbamazepine	50 µmol/l
Sodium valproate	600 µmol/l

*Primidone is metabolized in vivo largely to phenobarbitone.

IMMUNOLOGICAL INVESTIGATIONS

Assay	Normal value
Rheumatoid factor	
Latex screening	Positive/negative
Latex test	≤ 20
Sheep cell agglutination test (Rose–Waaler) (SCAT)	≤ 32
Differental agglutination test (DAT)	≤ 16
Antinuclear antibodies	≤ 10

SYNOVIAL FLUID ANALYSIS

	Normal	Osteoarthritis	Inflammatory	Septic	Crystal arthritis
Appearance	Clear, colourless	Clear, yellow	Cloudy/turbid; yellow/brown	Turbid; brown/green	Cloudy/turbid; yellow/brown
Viscosity	High	High	Low	Low	Low
Fibrin clot	Absent	Absent	Present	Present	Usually present
Cell count	$0.2–1 \times 10^9/l$	$0.2–5 \times 10^9/l$	$2–100 \times 10^9/l$	$20–100 \times 10^9/l$	$20–100 \times 10^9/l$
Special features	None	None	lupus erythematosis (LE) cells:? complement	Culture and inoculate into guinea pig	Crystals, uric acid, pyrophosphate

IMMUNOSPECIFICITIES OF ANTINUCLEAR ANTIBODIES

Immunospecificity	Disease
Antibodies to DNA	
Identical determinants on native and denatured DNA	High titre in systemic lupus erythematosus (SLE). Low titres in other rheumatic diseases
Single-strand (denatured) DNA-purine and pyrimidine determinants	Present in rheumatic and non-rheumatic diseases
Antibodies to histones	
H1, H2A, H2B, H3, H4	Present in 30% of patients with systemic lupus erythematosis (SLE), almost always in association with other antinuclear antibodies (ANAs). Present in 95% of procainamide induced LE as the only type of ANA
Antibodies to non-histone antigens	
Sm antigen	Marker antibody for SLE
Nuclear ribonucleoprotein (nRNP)	High titres in mixed connective tissue disease
SSA and SSB antigens	Common in Sjögren's syndrome; low titres in some other rheumatic diseases
Scl-70	Highly diagnostic of scleroderma
Centromere protein	Highly diagnostic of CRST syndrome/scleroderma
RA-associated nuclear antigen (RANA)	Present in RA and Sjögren's syndrome with RA
Proliferating cell nuclear antigen (PCNA)	Present in <10% of patients with SLE
Antibodies to nucleolar antigens	
4S–6S nucleolus-specific RNA	Present in patients with scleroderma or Raynaud's phenomenon
Other unidentified nucleolar antigens	Present in scleroderma or overlap diseases with features of scleroderma and/or Raynaud's phenomenon

Reprinted with permission from Tan EM. Significance of antinuclear antibodies. *Aust N Z J Med* (1981), **11**: 193–6.

**RIDDOR: REPORTABLE DISEASES FROM SCHEDULE
3 OF THE REGULATIONS**

1. Inflammation, ulceration or malignant disease of the skin due to ionizing radiation.
2. Malignant disease of the bones due to ionizing radiation
3. Blood dyscrasia due to ionizing radiation
4. Cataract due to electromagnetic radiation
5. Decompression illness
6. Barotrauma resulting in lung or other organ damage
7. Dysbaric osteonecrosis
8. Cramps of the hand or forearm due to repetitive movements
9. Subcutaneous cellulitis of the hand (beat hand)
10. Bursitis or subcutaneous cellulitis arising at or about the knee due to severe or prolonged external friction or pressure at or about the knee (beat knee)
11. Bursitis or subcutaneous cellulitis arising at or about the elbow due to severe or prolonged external friction or pressure at or about the elbow (beat elbow)
12. Traumatic inflammation of the tendons of the hand or forearm or of the associated tendon sheaths
13. Carpal tunnel syndrome
14. Hand-arm vibration syndrome
15. Anthrax
16. Brucellosis
17. (a) Avian chlamydiosis; (b) ovine chlamydiosis
18. Hepatitis
19. Legionellosis
20. Leptospirosis
21. Lyme disease
22. Q fever
23. Rabies
24. Streptococcus suis
25. Tetanus
26. Tuberculosis
27. Any infection reliably attributable to work with live or dead human beings, blood, body fluids, animals, micro-organisms or any other potentially infected material derived from them
28. Poisonings by any of the following:
    (a) acrylamide monomer
    (b) arsenic or one of its compounds
    (c) benzene or a homologue of benzene
    (d) beryllium or one of its compounds
    (e) cadmium or one of its compounds
    (f) carbon disulphide
    (g) diethylene dioxide (dioxan)
    (h) ethylene oxide
    (i) lead or one of its compounds
    (j) manganese or one of its compounds
    (k) mercury or one of its compounds
    (l) methyl bromide

- (m) nitrochlorobenzene, or a nitro- or amino- or chloro-derivative of benzene or of a homologue of benzene
- (n) oxides of nitrogen
- (o) phosphorus or one of its compounds
29 Cancer of a bronchus or lung
30 Primary carcinoma of the lung where there is accompanying evidence of silicosis
31 Cancer of the urinary tract
32 Bladder cancer
33 Angiocarcinoma of the liver
34 Peripheral neuropathy
35 Chrome ulceration of
- (a) the nose or throat or
- (b) the skin of the hands or forearm
36 Folliculitis
37 Acne
38 Skin cancer
39 Pneumoconiosis (excluding asbestosis)
40 Bysinosis
41 Mesothelioma
42 Lung cancer
43 Asbestosis
44 Cancer of the nasal cavity or associated air sinuses
45 Occupational dermatitis
46 Extrinsic alveolitis (including farmer's lung)
47 Occupational asthma

Note: Reporting of Injuries, Diseases and Dangerous Occurrences Regulations 1995 (RIDDOR) came into effect on 1 April 1996.

CLASSIFICATION OF DRUGS

Drugs	Used to
ACE inhibitors	Inhibit conversion of angiotensin I to angiotensin II
Alpha blockers	Antagonize noradrenaline vasoconstriction
Anaesthetics	Destroy sensibility
Analeptics	Stimulate respiration
Antacids	Neutralize gastric acidity
Anthelmintics	Destroy worms in alimentary tract
Antiamoebics	Treat amoebic dysentery and hepatitis
Antiarrhythmics	Restore cardiac rhythm
Antibiotics	Inhibit growth of micro-organisms
Anticholinergics	Block parasympathetic secretory responses
Anticoagulants	Increase blood clotting time
Anticonvulsants	Decrease motor activity
Antidepressants	Counteract depression
Antidiarrhoeals	Reduce diarrhoea
Antiemetics	Reduce vomiting
Antifungals	Destroy fungal cells

OCCUPATIONAL MEDICINE/ THERAPEUTICS

CLASSIFICATION OF DRUGS (cont'd)

Drugs	Used to
Antimalarials	Used for prophylaxis and treatment of malaria
Antihypertensives	Reduce blood pressure
Antipruritics	Relieve itching
Antipsychotics	Reduce psychotic symptoms
Antipyretics	Reduce temperature
Antiseptics	Prevent multiplication of micro-organisms
Antispasmodics	Relieve spasm of involuntary muscle
Antithyroid	Inhibit formation of thyroxin
Antitoxins	Neutralize bacterial toxins
Antivirals	Exert antiviral activity
Astringents	Precipitate proteins on skin surface
Anxiolitics	Reduce anxiety
Beta blockers	Decrease sympathetic effect of cardiovascular system
Bronchodilators	Relax airway smooth muscle
Calcium agonists	Cause coronary vasodilation
Carminatives	Relieve flatulence
Cholagogues	Increase flow of bile
Contraceptives	Prevent conception
Cytoprotectants	Enhance secretion of mucus
Diaphoretics	Increase sweating
Disinfectants	Destroy micro-organisms
Diuretics	Increase urinary output
Ecbolics	Stimulate uterine contractions
Emetics	Produce vomiting
Expectorants	Stimulate bronchial secretion
Fibrinolytics	Produce thrombolysis
5 HT Re-uptake inhibitors	Block neurotransmitters
Fungicides	Inhibit fungal growth
Haematinics	Treat anaemia
Haemostatics	Reduce bleeding
H$_2$ Receptor antagonists	Reduce gastric acid secretion
Hypnotics	Induce sleep
Hypoglycaemic agents	Reduce blood sugar
Hypolipidaemic agents	Reduce hyperlipoproteinaemia
Immunosuppressants	Prevent transplant rejection
Laxatives	Ease constipation
Miotics	Contract the pupil
Muscle relaxants	Relax smooth muscle
Mydriatics	Dilate the pupil
Narcotics	Induce sleep and relieve pain
Non steroidal anti-inflammatory drugs	Reduce inflammation
Oestrogen receptor antagonists	Treat breast cancer
Proton pump inhibitors	Inhibit gastric secretion
Purgatives	Stimulate bowel action
Sedatives	Reduce activity of nervous system
Stimulants	Increase activity of nervous system
Tonics	Improve the appetite
Tranquillizers	Reduce nervous tension
Vaccines	Immunize against infectious diseases

DRUGS AND DOSAGES

Generic name	Average single adult dose by mouth	Proprietary name
Acetylsalicylic acid	300 mg	Aspirin
Acyclovir	200 mg	Zovirax
Alendronate sodium	10 mg	Fosamax
Allopurinol	300 mg	Zyloric
Aluminium hydrox	475 mg	Alu-cap
Amiloride hydrochloride	5 mg	Moduretic
Amitriptyline	25 mg	Tryptizol
Amlodipine	5 mg	Istin
Amoxycillin	250 mg	Amoxil
Atenolol	100 mg	Tenormin
Azathioprine	25 mg	Imuran
Beclomethasone dipropionate	50 µg inhalation	Becotide
Bendrofluazide	5 mg	Aprinox
Benzylpenicillin	250 mg	Crystapen G
Betamethasone	500 µg	Betnesol
Bisacodyl	5 mg	Dulcolax
Bisoprolol	10 mg	Monocor
Bisphosphonate alendronate	10 mg	Fosamax
Captopril	25 mg	Capoten
Carbamazepine	100 mg	Tegretol
Cefaclor	375 mg	Distaclor
Cefuroxine axetil	250 mg	Zinnat
Chlorambucil	2 mg	Leukeran
Chloroquine	250 mg	Avloclor
Chlorpheniramine maleate	4 mg	Piriton
Chlorpromazine hydrochloride	25 mg	Largactil
Cimetidine	400 mg	Tagamet
Ciprofloxin	250 mg	Ciproxin
Cyanocobalamin	250 µg im	Cytamen
Cyclosporin	50 mg	Sandimmun
Diamorphine hydrochloride	10 mg	Heroin
Diazepam	5 mg	Valium
Diclofenac sodium	25 mg	Voltarol
Dihydrocodeine	30 mg	DF 118
Digoxin	250 µg	Lanoxin
Diltiazem	200 mg	Tildiem
Disopyramide	100 mg	Rythmodan
Domperidone	10 mg	Motilium
Dothiepin hydrochloride	75 mg	Prothiaden
Enalapril	5 mg	Innovace
Ergometrine maleate	500 µg	Syntometrine
Ergotamine tartrate	2 mg (sub ling.)	Lingraine
Ephedrine hydrochloride	30 mg	C.A.M.
Erythromycin	250 mg	Erythrocin
Ethinyloestradiol	50 µg	
Ferrous sulphate	150 mg	Ferrograd
Finasteride	5 mg	Proscar
Fluoxitine	20 mg	Prozac
Fluticaone proprionate	100 mg inhalation	Flixotide
Flucloxacillin	250 mg	Floxapen
Folic acid	5 mg	
Frusemide	40 mg	Lasix
Gliclazide	80 mg	Diamicron
Hyoscine butylbromide	10 mg	Buscopan
Ibuprofen	400 mg	Brufen
Imipramine	10 mg	Tofranil
Indomethacin	25 mg	Indocid
Isoniazid	25 mg (im)	Rimifon
Isosorbide mononitrate	60 mg	Imdur

DRUGS AND DOSAGES (cont'd)

Generic name	Average single adult dose by mouth	Proprietary name
Isoprenaline sulphate	400 µg (inhaler)	Medihaler-Iso
Ketoconazole	200 mg	Nizoral
Ketoprofen	250 mg	Orudis
Lactulose	3.5 g/5 ml	Duphalac
Lansoprazole	15 mg	Zoton
Levodopa	50 mg	Sinemet
Lisinopril	10 mg	Zestril
Loperamide hydrochloride	2 mg	Imodium
Lorazepam	1 mg	Ativan
Mebendazole	100 mg	Vermox
Mebeverine	135 mg	Colofac
Mefenamic acid	500 mg	Ponstan
Methadone hydrochloride	5 mg	Physeptone
Metformin	500 mg	Glucophage
Metoclopramide	10 mg	Maxolon
Metronidazole	200 mg	Flagyl
Morphine sulphate	10 mg (sc/im)	
Nalidixic acid	500 mg	Negram
Naproxen	250 mg	Naprosyn
Nicardipine	20 mg	Cardene
Nifedipine	10 mg	Adalat
Nitrazepam	5 mg	Mogadon
Norethisterone	5 mg	Primolut N
Omeprazole	20 mg	Losec
Oxprenolol hydrochloride	20 mg	Trasicor
Oxybutynin	5 mg	Ditropan
Oxytetracycline	250 mg	Terramycin
Oxytocin	1 U/l (iv)	Syntocinon
Paracetamol	500 mg	Panadol
Paroxetine	20 mg	Seroxat
Pethidine hydrochloride	100 mg (im)	
Phenobarbitone	30 mg	Luminal
Phenytoin sodium	100 mg	Epanutin
Piroxicam	10 mg	Feldene
Potassium chloride	600 mg	Slow K
Prednisolone	5 mg	Prednesol
Procaine penicillin	300 mg (im)	Depocillin
Proguanil hydrochloride	100 mg	Paludrine
Prochlorperazine	5 mg	Stemetil
Procyclidine	5 mg	Kemadrin
Promethazine hydrochloride	25 mg	Phenergan
Propanolol hydrochloride	80 mg	Inderal
Quinine bisulphate	300 mg	
Ranitidine	150 mg	Zantac
Rifampicin	300 mg	Rifadin
Simvastatin	10 mg	Zocor
Sodium cromoglycate	1 mg (inhalation)	Intal
Stilboestrol	5 mg	Apstil
Sumatriptan	50 mg	Imigran
Tamoxifen	10 mg	Nolvadex
Temazepam	10 mg	Temazepam
Terfenadine	60 mg	Triludan
Testosterone propionate	25 mg (im)	Virormone
Tiaprofenic acid	300 mg	Surgam SA
Thioridazine	25 mg	Melleril
Thyroxine sodium	50 µg	Eltroxin
Tolbutamide	500 mg	Rastinon
Tramadol hydrochloride	100 mg	Zydol
Trimethoprim	200 mg	Septrin
Zopiclone	7.5 mg	Zimovane

ANTI-ASTHMATIC DRUGS

β_2 sympathomimetic drugs
  Salbutamol (Ventolin), terbutaline (Bricanyl). Can be given systemically or by inhalation. Effective during bronchospasm. Action is rapid especially if inhaled

Xanthines
  Aminophylline, choline theophyllinate, or slow release aminophylline (e.g. phyllocontin). Used systemically. Effective during bronchospasm. Also have a useful prophylactic effect

Sodium cromoglycate (Intal)
  Inhalation only. No good in established bronchospasm; prophylactic only. Very low toxicity

Steroid group
  Systemic
    Using oral or injected steroids such as prednisolone or hydrocortisone. Effective during bronchospasm. Powerful, but slow onset of action. Any of the steroid side-effects may occur if used long term. Poor growth is the most important in children; may be less with alternate day administration
  Inhaled
    Such as beclomethasone dipropionate (Becotide), betamethasone valerate (Bextasol) Fluticasone Propionate (Flixotide). No good if bronchospasm present; prophylactic only; very effective

Anticholinergic drugs
  Ipratropium (Atrovent) effective bronchodilator. Useful in toddlers. A few older children respond better to it than the sympathomimetic drugs (Reiser and Warner, 1986). Can be combined with salbutamol, but not in severe attacks (Lenney and Storr, 1986).

Antihistamines
  Pretty useless in children

From Lenney W, Storr J (1986) Nebulized ipratropium and salbutamol in asthma Archives of Diseases in Childhood, 54:116–119. Published in Modell M, Boyd R Paediatric Problems in General Practice, 2nd edn, Oxford Medical Publications
From Reiser J, Warner J O (1986) Inhalation Treatment for Asthma, Archives of Diseases of Childhood, 61:88–94. Published in Modell M, Boyd R Paediatric Problems in General Practice, 2nd edn, Oxford Medical Publications

POTENCY OF STEROID PREPARATIONS

Weak preparations (potency IV)
  Hydrocortisone 0.5, 1 or 2.5% — nothing stronger than this should be used on the face

Intermediate preparations (potency III)
  Flurandrenolone 0.0125% (Haelan); clobetasone butyrate 0.05% (Eumovate); betamethasone 0.025% (Betnovate-RD); Alphaderm (1% hydrocortisone with urea)

Strong preparations (potency II)
  Betamethasone 0.1% (Betnovate); flucinolone acetonide 0.025% (Synalar); beclomethasone dipropionate 0.025% (Propaderm)

Very strong preparations (potency I)
  Clobetasol propionate 0.05% (Dermovate); flucinolone acetonide 0.2% (Synalar Forte)

DRUGS FOR ACUTE MEDICAL EMERGENCIES

Drug	Use	Dosage
Adrenaline (1 mg/ml) 1 in 1000	Anaphylaxis or acute angio-oedema	Give intramuscularly or subcutaneously Adults 0.5–1 ml 6–12 year olds 0.5 ml* 5 year olds 0.4 ml* 3–4 year olds 0.3 ml* 2 year olds 0.2 ml* 1 year olds 0.1 ml Under 1 year 0.05 ml Repeat every 10 min if necessary
Amoxycillin (250 mg vial)	Severe pneumonia in a patient with chronic respiratory disease	500 mg intramuscularly or intravenously
Atropine (600 µg/ml)	Bradycardia and hypotension associated with myocardial infarction	300 µg intravenously, increasing to 1 mg as necessary
Benzylpenicillin (600 mg vial)	Suspected meningococcal disease	Give intramuscularly or intravenously Infants under 1 year 300 mg Children 1–9 years 600 mg Older children and adults 1200 mg
Chlorpheniramine (10 mg/ml)	As an adjunct to adrenaline to prevent relapse in the treatment of anaphylaxis or acute angio-oedema	10–20 mg, intravenously (over 1–2 minutes), diluted with 10 ml of the patient's blood drawn back into the syringe or with sterile sodium chloride 0.9% or water for injection
Chlorpromazine (25 mg/ml)	Agitated psychotic patients	25–50 mg by deep intramuscular injection
Cyclizine (50 mg/ml)	Vomiting due to vestibular disorders or with diamorphine	50 mg intramuscularly or intravenously
Diamorphine (5 or 10 mg powder in vials, plus an ampoule of water for injection for reconstitution of powder)	Severe pain (e.g. myocardial infarction)	5 mg by slow intravenous injection, as 1 mg/minute, followed by a further 2.5–5 mg if necessary
	Acute left heart failure	2.5–5 mg by slow intravenous injection, as 1 mg/minute
Diazepam (5 mg/ml as Diazemuls)	Severe acute anxiety and panic attacks when alternative measures have failed or tablets are inappropriate	10 mg by slow intravenous injection (5 mg/min) into a large vein, or intramuscularly if an intravenous route cannot be established
Flumazenil (100 µg/ml)	To reverse any respiratory depression caused by parenteral diazepam (as above)	200 µg intravenously over 15 s, then 100 µg at 60 s intervals if required, up to a maximum of 1 mg
Frusemide (10 mg/ml)	Relief of pulmonary oedema associated with left heart failure	20–50 mg intravenously, at a maximum rate of 4 mg/min
Glucagon (1 mg/ml)	Hypoglycaemia (as an alternative to glucose)	0.5–1 mg subcutaneously, intramuscularly or intravenously (NB if no response after 15 min give intravenous glucose as below)
Glucose solution (50 ml vial of 50%)	Hypoglycaemia when patient is unconscious	Up to 50 ml as an intravenous infusion
Haloperidol (5 mg/ml)	Agitated psychotic patients	2–10 mg intramuscularly every 4–8 h (or every hour if necessary)
Hydrocortisone (100 mg powder as sodium succinate for reconstitution with water for injection)	To prevent further deterioration in patients severely affected by an anaphylactic reaction	100–300 mg intravenously after adrenaline
	Acute asthma attack	200 mg (children 100 mg) by intravenous injection over at least 30–60 s
Metoclopramide (5 mg/ml)	Vomiting	10 mg intramuscularly or intravenously over 1–2 min
Naloxone (400 µg/ml)	Opioid overdose	800 µg–2 mg intravenously, which can be repeated every 2–3 min up to 10 mg if there is no response
Prochlorperazine (12.5 mg/ml)	Vomiting	12.5 mg by deep intramuscular injection

*Suitable for robust children. For underweight children, use half these doses.

DRUG INTERACTIONS: POTENTIALLY LETHAL COMBINATIONS*

Primary drug	Interactant
Adrenaline	Chloroform
	Cyclopropane
	Fl[uroxene
	Halothane
	Methoxyflurane
	Sympathomimetic drugs (status asthmaticus)
Alcohol	Acetaldehyde dehydrogenase inhibitors (disulfiram, etc.)
	Barbiturates
	Chloral hydrate
	Insulin
	Meprobamate
	Methotrexate
	Morphine and narcotic analgesics
	Muscle relaxants
	Nitrates and nitrites
	Sedatives and hypnotics
	Tricyclic antidepressants
Amitriptyline	Guanethidine
Amphetamines	MAO inhibitors
Anaesthetics	Adrenergic neuron blockers
	Antibiotics (with neuromuscular blocking action)
	Barbiturates
	Catecholamines
	Corticosteroids
	Kanamycin
	MAO inhibitors
	Neomycin
	Propranolol
	Sedatives and hypnotics
Antibiotics (with neuromuscular blocking action) (bacitracin, dihydrostreptomycin gentamycin, gramicidin, kanamycin, neomycin, polymyxin B, streptomycin, viomycin, etc.)	Anaesthetics
	Antibiotics (with neuromuscular blocking action)
	Muscle relaxants
Anticoagulants (coumarin, warfarin, etc.)	Analgesics (aspirin, pyrazolones, etc.)
	Clofibrate
	Dextrothyroxine
	Indomethacin
	Oxyphenbutazone
	Phenylbutazone
	Salicylates
	Thyroid preparations
Anticonvulsants	Methylphenidate

*With high dosage, or in susceptible patient.

THERAPEUTICS 49

**DRUG INTERACTIONS: POTENTIALLY LETHAL
COMBINATIONS* (cont'd)**

Primary drug	Interactant
Antidepressants (tricyclic)	Alcohol
	Diphenylhydantoin
	Guanethidine
	MAO inhibitors
	Reserpine
Antidiabetics (oral)	MAO inhibitors
Antihistamines	CNS depressants (barbiturates, etc.)
Antineoplastics	Attenuated live virus vaccines
Appetite suppressants (sympathomimetic)	MAO inhibitors
Caffeine (in excess)	MAO inhibitors
Carbamazepine	MAO inhibitors
Catecholamines	Anaesthetics (chloroform, ether, etc.)
	Guanethidine
Cheese (ripe, strong)	MAO inhibitors
Chicken livers	MAO inhibitors
Chloral hydrate	Alcohol
Chloramphenicol	Anticoagulants (oral)
	Antidiabetics (oral)
Chloroform	Catecholamines
Clofibrate	Anticoagulants (oral)
Colistimethate	Antibiotics (with neuromuscular blocking action)
	Muscle relaxants (peripherally acting)
Corticosteroids	Anaesthetics
	Vaccines (live, attenuated)
Curariform drugs	Antibiotics (with neuromuscular blocking action)
	Furosemide
	Quinidine
Cyclopropane	Adrenaline
	Levarterenol
Dextromethorphan	MAO inhibitors (phenelzine, etc.)
Dextrothyroxine	Anticoagulants (oral)
Digitalis	Calcium salts (iv)
	Diuretics (hypokalaemia)
	Propranolol
Diphenylhydantoin	Disulfiram
	Folic acid antagonists (methotrexate, etc.)
	Phenyramidol
	Sulphonamides
Disulfiram	Alcohol
Dopa	MAO inhibitors
Ephedrine	MAO inhibitors
Ethacrynic acid	Anticoagulants (oral)
Ether	Neomycin
	Propranolol
Furosemide	Muscle relaxants
Guanethidine	Antidepressants
	MAO inhibitors
Insulin	Alcohol

DRUG INTERACTIONS: POTENTIALLY LETHAL COMBINATIONS* (cont'd)

Primary drug	Interactant
Isoproterenol	Adrenaline
	MAO inhibitors
Kanamycin	Anaesthetics
	Antibiotics (with neuromuscular blocking action)
	Muscle relaxants
	Procainamide
Levarterenol	Anaesthetics (halogenated, cyclopropane, etc.)
	Antidepressants (tricyclic)
	Guanethidine
MAO inhibitors	Amphetamines
	Anaesthetics
	Antidepressants
	(MAO inhibitors, tricyclics)
	Antidiabetics (oral)
	Caffeine (excessive amounts)
	Carbamazepine
	Cheese (ripe, strong)
	CNS depressants
	Dextromethorphan
	Ephedrine
	Guanethidine
	Isoproterenol
	Levodopa
	Liver (beef/chicken)
	Meperidine
	Methyldopa
	Methylphenidate
	Propranolol
	Reserpine
	Sympathomimetic appetite suppressants
	Tyramine-rich foods
Meperidine	MAO inhibitors
Methotrexate	Sulphonamides
Methyldopa	MAO inhibitors
Muscle relaxants	Anaesthetics (halogenated)
(depolarizing)	Antibiotics (with neuromuscular blocking action)
Nitrates/nitrites	Alcohol
Quinidine	Muscle relaxants
Reserpine	Antidepressants
	Digitalis
	MAO inhibitors
Salicylates	Anticoagulants (oral)
Sedatives/hypnotics	Alcohol
	Antidepressants
Sulphonamides	Antidiabetics (oral)
(long-acting)	Diphenylhydantoin
	Folic acid antagonists
	Methotrexate
Tetracyclines	Aluminium-containing antacids
	Methoxyflurane
Ticrynafen	Diphenylhydantoin
	Warfarin

THERAPEUTICS 51

SUSCEPTIBILITY OF SELECTED BACTERIA TO CERTAIN ANTIBACTERIAL DRUGS

Bacterium	Penicillin V/G	Flucloxacillin	Amp/amoxycillin	Carbenicillin/ticarcillin	Piperacillin/azlocillin/mezlocillin	Cephradine/cephalothin/cefazolin	Cefuroxime/cephamandole/cefotaxime	Ceftazidime	Erythromycin	Lincomycin/clindamycin	Tetracyclines	Chloramphenicol	Trimethoprim	Aminoglycosides	Vancomycin	Metronidazole
Staphylococcus aureus (penicillin sensitive)	1	1	0	0	0	2	2	0	2R	R	2R	R	R	2	2	R
Staphylococcus aureus (penicillin resistant)	R	1	R	R	R	R	R	R	R	R	2R	R	R	R	2	R
Streptococcus (group A)	1	0	0	0	0	2	2	0	2R	R	R	R	R	2R	2	R
Streptococcus pneumoniae	1	0	1	0	0	2	2	0	2R	R	R	R	R	R	0	R
Streptococcus faecalis	2	0	1	0	2	R	R	R	0	0	R	R	R	R	0	R
Neisseria meningitidis	1	0	0	0	0	0	0	0	0	0	0	2	0	R	2R	R
Listeria monocytogenes	2	R	2	R	R	R	2	R	R	R	R	2	R	R	0	R
Haemophilus influenzae	R	R	1R	R	R	2	2	2	R	R	2R	R	1R	2	R	R
Escherichia coli	R	R	R	R	R	2	2	2	R	R	R	R	1R	0	R	R
Klebsiella spp.	R	R	R	R	R	2	2	2	R	R	R	R	1R	2R	R	R
Serratia/Enterobacter spp.	R	R	R	R	R	R	2R	2R	R	R	R	R	1R	2R	R	R
Proteus spp.	R	R	R	R	R	2	2	2	R	R	R	R	R	1R	R	R
Pseudomonas aeruginosa	R	R	R	1R	1R	R	2R	2R	R	R	R	R	R	2R	R	R
Bacteroides fragilis	R	R	R	R	R	R	R	R	2R	2R	2R	2R	R	R	R	1
Other bacteroides spp.	R	R	R	R	R	R	R	R	2R	2R	2R	2R	R	R	R	1

1, Susceptible, first choice; 2, susceptible, second choice; R, resistance likely to be a problem; 0, usually inappropriate.

IV FLUID THERAPY IN DEHYDRATION

	Clinical assessment	Laboratory aids
Volume losses	Signs of dehydration	PCV
	Signs of shock	Blood urea
Osmolar changes	Hypernatraemia	
	Irritability	Plasma Na^+
	Skin 'doughy'	Plasma osmolality
	Circulation relatively good	
	Hyponatraemia	Plasma Na^+
	Shock	Plasma osmolality (high
	Hypotension	urine osmolality suggests inappropriate ADH secretion)
Acid–base	Hyperpnoea	Blood gases, pH, HCO_3^- bicarbonate
	Tachypnoea	
Loss of intracellular cation (K^+)	Weakness	Plasma K^+
	Hypotonia	ECG changes reflect plasma level
Hypocalcaemia	Neuromuscular irritability	Total plasma calcium not a good guide; ionized calcium ideal; ECG changes helpful
Hypoglycaemia	Lethargy	Blood sugar
	Coma	
	Convulsion	

PRINCIPLES OF ELECTROLYTE REPLACEMENT

Principle
    Total fluid requirements = maintenance + 0.2 normal saline in 4.3%
                                                  glucose plus KCI
                                                            +
                                              deficit + normal saline plus KCI
                                                            +
                                          ongoing loss normal saline plus KCI

Action		
0–1/2 h	Treat shock immediately	Plasma or normal saline 20 ml/kg body weight
1/2–4 h	Initial replacement (awaiting serum electrolyte results)	0.5 normal or normal saline 10 ml/kg/h
4–24 h	Continuing replacement	
	If serum Na below 150 mmol/l	0.2 normal saline in 4.3% dextrose plus KCI 30–40 mmol/l and plan total correction over 24 h
	If serum Na above 150 mmol/l	0.2 normal saline in 4.3% dextrose plus KCI 30–40 mmol/l. Restrict fluids to 150 ml/kg in first 24 h and plan total correction over 48 h

COMMONLY USED IV FLUIDS AND DRUGS

Solution (abbreviation)	Concentration (mmol/l)					Energy content	
	Na	Cl	K	Ca	Bic	Glucose	(Cal/l)
IV Fluids							
Normal saline (NaCl 0.9%)	150	150	—	—	—	—	—
1/2 normal saline + Dextrose (NaCl 0.45% Dextrose 5%)	77	77	—	—	—	28	180
1/5 normal saline + Dextrose (NaCl 0.18% Dextrose 4%)	30	30	—	—	—	22.4	150
1/2 strength Hartmann's solution (1/2 strength H)	66	56	3	1	14	—	—
1/2 strength Hartmann's solution (1/2 strength H + Dextrose 5%) and Dextrose	66	56	3	1	14	28	180

IV drugs
    Sodium bicarbonate 8.4% solution: 1 ml contains 1 mmol sodium bicarbonate
    Potassium chloride 20% solution: 5 ml contains 13 mmol K (= 1 g)
    Calcium gluconate 10% solution: 10 ml contains 2.25 mmol Ca 2

Burettes for IV fluids: Soluset: ml/h = drops/min Hemoset (for blood administration): ml/h = (drops/min).

NORMAL FLUID BALANCE

In	Volume (ml)	Out	Volume (ml)
Oral fluids	1500	Insensible loss	
Water from solid food	600	Faeces	200
Water of oxidation (20 ml/420 J)	300	Lungs	400
		Skin	400
		Sweat (temperate climate)	200
		Urine	1200
Total	2400	Total	2400

ELECTROLYTE CONCENTRATIONS — INTRAVENOUS FLUIDS

Intravenous infusion	mmol/l				
	Na$^+$	K$^+$	HCO$_3^-$	Cl$^-$	Ca^{2+}
Normal plasma values	142	4.5	26	103	2.5
Sodium chloride 0.9%	150	—	—	150	—
Compound sodium lactate (Hartmann's)	131	5	29	111	2
Sodium chloride 0.18% and glucose 4%	30	—	—	30	—
Potassium chloride 0.3% and glucose 5%	—	40	—	40	—
Potassium chloride 0.3% and Sodium chloride 0.9%	150	40	—	190	—
To correct metabolic acidosis					
Sodium bicarbonate 1.26%	150	—	150	—	—
Sodium bicarbonate	1000	—	1000	—	—
8.4% for cardiac arrest					
Sodium lactate (M/6)	167	—	167	—	—

MILLIMOLES OF EACH ION IN 1 G SALT

Electrolyte	mmol/g approx.
Ammonium chloride	18.7
Calcium chloride	Ca: 6.8
($CaCl_2.2H_2O$)	Cl: 13.6
Potassium bicarbonate	10
Potassium chloride	13.4
Sodium bicarbonate	11.9
Sodium chloride	17.1
Sodium lactate	8.9

ELECTROLYTE CONTENT — GASTROINTESTINAL SECRETIONS

Type of fluid	mmol/l				
	H^+	Na^+	K^+	HCO_3^-	Cl^-
Gastric	40–60	20–80	5–20	—	100–150
Biliary	—	120–140	5–15	30–50	80–120
Pancreatic	—	120–140	5–15	70–110	40–80
Small bowel	—	120–140	5–15	20–40	90–130

Faeces, vomit or aspiration should be saved and analysed where possible
if abnormal losses are suspected; where this is impracticable these
approximations may be helpful in planning replacement treatment.

FLOW-RATE/INFUSION TIME

Calculation formulae:

$$\text{Flow-rate (drops per minute)} = \frac{\text{Drops in 1 ml} \times \text{total (ml)}}{\text{Total time (min)}}$$

$$\text{Infusion time} = \frac{\text{Total vol. to be delivered}}{\text{ml being delivered per hour}}$$

BLOOD TRANSFUSION: BLOOD GROUPS

Group	Frequency % (white faces)	Red cells			Serum	
		Agglutinated by serum of group	Contain agglutinogen	Transfused from donor of	Agglutinates cells of	Contains agglutinin
AB	5	O, A, B	A, B	A, B, AB, O	None	None
A	40	O, B	A	A or O	AB, B	b
B	10	O, A	B	B or O	AB, A	a
O	45	None	None	O	AB, A, B	a, b
Rh +ve	86			Rh +ve or −ve		
Rh −ve	14			Rh −ve		

1 Effect of patient's serum on donor's red cells is of importance — not reverse.
2 Donor's blood tested directly against serum of patient for compatibility and against sera of known A and known B groups.
3 *Emergency* only group O, Rh negative blood may be used — 'Universal Donor'.

BLOOD TRANSFUSION: LABORATORY INVESTIGATIONS

Incorrectly or incompletely labelled samples/request forms will not be accepted. **Full identification is absolutely necessary.**

Investigation	Result	Sample
Group and save serum/cross match	—	May be done on one 10 ml clotted sample, special BT tube. Take a second sample into lithium heparin if patient is receiving heparin treatment
		Consult lab.
Cold agglutinin titres		EDTA sample
DCT direct Coombs test	Negative	Consult lab. Suspect blood donation must be returned to the lab. together with EDTA sample and one 10 ml clotted sample, special BT tube
Transfusion reaction investigations		
Platelet antibodies	Negative	Consult lab.

SURGICAL PROCEDURES

Abdominal paracentesis	Evaluation of ascitic fluid
Adenectomy	Removal of glands
Angiography	Visualization of an artery with radio-opaque material
Angioplasty	Insertion and inflation of balloon-tipped catheter into coronary artery
Appendicectomy	Removal of appendix
Biopsy	Removal of tissue from the body for microscopic examination and diagnosis
Bronchial lavage	Installation of fluid into a lung
Bronchoscopy	Visual examination of the tracheobronchial tree
Cholecystectomy	Removal of gall bladder
Cholecystostomy	Opening and draining of gall bladder
Choledochotomy	Opening of the bile duct
Circumcision	Removal of the foreskin
Colonoscopy	Visual examination of lower intestinal tract
Colostomy	Making an opening into the colon
Curettage	Scraping the lining of the uterus
Enterostomy	Making an opening into the small intestine
Episiotomy	Incision of the perineum
Gastrectomy	Removal of part of the stomach
Gastroenterostomy	Making an opening between the stomach and small intestine
Gastrointestinal endoscopy	Visual examination of upper intestinal tract
Gastrojejunostomy	Making an opening between the stomach and jejunum
Gastrostomy	Making an opening between the stomach and the abdominal wall
Glossectomy	Removal of the tongue
Herniorrhaphy	Repair of a hernial orifice
Herniotomy	Removal of the hernia sac
Hysterectomy	Removal of the uterus
Ileostomy	Making an opening into the ileum
Laminectomy	Removal of part of the vertebra
Laparoscopy	Evaluation of intra-abdominal or pelvic pathology
Lithotrity	Crushing of a stone in the bladder
Lobectomy	Removal of a lobe
Mastectomy	Removal of the breast
Mediastinoscopy	Examination of the mediastinum through a scope
Mediastiotomy	Examination of the mediastinum through a parasternal incision
Menisectomy	Removal of a semi-lunar cartilage (in knee joint)
Nephrectomy	Removal of a kidney
Orchidectomy	Removal of a testicle

SURGICAL PROCEDURES (cont'd)

Osteotomy	Cutting a bone
Oophorectomy	Removal of an ovary
Perineorrhaphy	Suturing the perineum
Prostatectomy	Removal of the prostate
Retrograde pyelogram	Introduction of radio-opaque material directly into urinary tract
Salpingectomy	Removal of the fallopian tube
Saphenous ligation	Tying the saphenous vein
Sidmoidoscopy and anoscopy	Visual examination of perianal and distal rectum
Suprapubic cystotomy	Making an opening above the pubis into the bladder
Sympathectomy	Cutting of some of the sympathetic nerves
Tenotomy	Cutting of a tendon
Thoracoplasty	Removal of a rib to collapse a lung
Thoracotomy	Making an opening in the thoracic wall
Thyroidectomy	Removal of the thyroid gland
Tracheotomy	Making an opening into the trachea
Transplantation	Transferring living tissue or cells from one subject to another
Transurethral resection of the prostate (TURP)	Removal of portion of the prostate via the urethra
Trephining	Cutting a hole in the skull
Valcotomy	Incision of a heart valve

ABDOMINAL INCISIONS AND ABDOMINAL AREAS

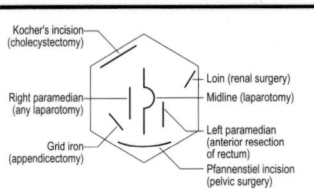

Kocher's incision (cholecystectomy)
Loin (renal surgery)
Right paramedian (any laparotomy)
Midline (laparotomy)
Grid iron (appendicectomy)
Left paramedian (anterior resection of rectum)
Pfannenstiel incision (pelvic surgery)

Abdominal areas

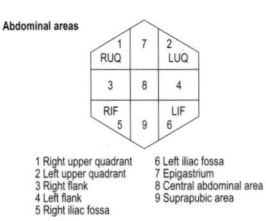

	1	7	2	
	RUQ		LUQ	
	3	8	4	
	RIF		LIF	
	5	9	6	

1 Right upper quadrant   6 Left iliac fossa
2 Left upper quadrant   7 Epigastrium
3 Right flank   8 Central abdominal area
4 Left flank   9 Suprapubic area
5 Right iliac fossa

ABBREVIATIONS USED IN PRESCRIPTIONS

Abbreviation	Latin	English
à. à.	Ana (Greek)	Of each
a.c.	Ante cibos	Before food
ad lib.	Ad libitum	As much as desired
alt. dieb.	Alternis diebus	Alternate days
alt. horis	Alternis horis	Alternate hours
alt. noct.	Alternis noctibus	Alternate nights
aq.	Aqua	Water
aq. dest.	Aqua destillata	Distilled water
aq. ster.	Aqua sterilisata	Sterile water
b.i.d. (b.d.)	Bis in die	Twice a day
B. P.	—	British Pharmacopoeia
c.	Cum	With
c.c.	Cum cibis	With food
c.m.	Cras mane	Tomorrow morning
c.n.	Cras nocte	Tomorrow night
co.	Compositum	Compound
dieb. alt.	Diebus alternis	On alternate days
dil.	Dilue	Dilute
f. or ft.	Fiat	Let it be made
h.n.	Hac nocte	Tonight
h.s.	Hora somni	At bedtime
in aq.	In aqua	In water
in d.	In dies	Daily
m.	Misce	Mix
man.	Mane	In the morning
m.d.u.	ut a me dictum	As directed by me
μg	—	micrograms
mit.	Mittee	Send
N. or Noct.	Nocte	At night
N. B.	Nota bene	Note well
n. et m.	Nocte et mane	Night and morning
N. F.	—	National Formulary
o.m.	Omni mane	Every morning
o.n.	Omni nocte	Every night
part. aeq.	Partes aequales	Equal parts
p.c.	Post cibos	After meals
p.o.	Per orum	By mouth
p.r.	Per rectum	By the rectum
p.r.n.	Pro re nata	As occasion arises
p.v.	Per vaginam	By the vagina
q.d. or q.i.d.	Quarter in die	Four times a day
q.d.s.	Quarter die sumendum	To be taken four times a day
q.h.	Quaque hora	Every hour
q. 4h.	Quarta quaque hora	Every four hours
q.l.	Quantum libet	As much as wanted
q.s.	Quantum sufficiat	A sufficient quantity
quotid	Quotidie	Daily
R.	Recipe	Take
rep.	Repetatur	Let it be repeated
rep. sem.	Repetatut Semel	Let it be repeated once
sig.	Signetur	Let it be labelled
sine	Sine	Without
s.o.s.	Si opus sit	If necessary
s.s.	Semis	A half
stat.	Statim	Immediately
t.d. or t.i.d.	Ter in die	Three times a day
t.d.s.	Ter die sumendum	To be given three times daily
ut dict.	ut dictum	As directed

MEDICAL ABBREVIATIONS IN GENERAL USAGE

▶	This is important
▶▶	Prompt action
♂/♀	Male to female ratio
~	Approximately
−ve	Negative
+ve	Positive
↓	Decreased
↑	Increased
↔	Normal
ABPA	Allergic bronchopulmonary aspergillosis
ACE	Angiotensin converting enzyme
ACTH	Adrenocorticotrophic hormone
ADH	Antidiuretic hormone
AF	Atrial fibrillation
AFB	Acid-fast bacillus
AIDS	Acquired immunodeficiency syndrome
Alk phos	Alkaline phosphatase
AMP	Adenosine monophosphate
ANF	Antinuclear factor
ARDS	Adult respiratory distress syndrome
ASD	Atrial septal defect
ASO	Antistreptolysin O
AST	Aspartate transaminase
ATN	Acute tubular necrosis
AV	Atrioventricular
AXR	Abdominal X-ray (plain)
Ba	Barium
BCR	British comparative ratio (= INR)
BMJ	*British Medical Journal*
BNF	*British National Formulary*
BP	Blood pressure
Ca	Carcinoma
cAMP	Cyclic AMP
CBD	Common bile duct
CCF	Congestive cardiac failure (i.e. RVF with LVF)
CI	Contraindications
CK	Creatine kinase
CLL	Chronic lymphocytic leukaemia
CML	Chronic myeloid leukaemia
CMV	Cytomegalovirus
CNS	Central nervous system
COAD	Chronic obstructive airway disease
CRF	Chronic renal failure
CSF	Cerebrospinal fluid
CT	Computed tomography
CVP	Central venous pressure
CVS	Cardiovascular system
CXR	Chest X-ray
DIC	Disseminated intravascular coagulation
DIP	Distal interphalangeal
DoH	Department of Health
DM	Diabetes mellitus
D&V	Diarrhoea and vomiting
DVT	Deep venous thrombosis
DXT	Deep radiotherapy
EBV	Epstein–Barr virus
ECG	Electrocardiogram
EEG	Electroencephalogram
EM	Electron microscope
ENT	Ear, nose and throat
ESR	Erythrocyte sedimentation rate
FBC	Full blood count
FEV_1	Forced expiratory volume in one second

MEDICAL ABBREVIATIONS IN GENERAL USAGE
(cont'd)

FFP	Fresh frozen plasma
F$_i$O$_2$	Partial pressure of O$_2$ in inspired air
FSH	Follicle-stimulating hormone
FVC	Forced vital capacity
GB	Gall bladder
GC	Gonococcus
GFR	Glomerular filtration rate
GH	Growth hormone
GI	Gastrointestinal
GP	General practitioner
G6PD	Glucose 6-phosphate dehydrogenase
GU	Genitourinary
Hb	Haemoglobin
HBsAg	Hepatitis B surface antigen
Hct	Haematocrit
HIDA	Hepatic immunodiacetic acid
HIV	Human immunodeficiency virus
HOCM	Hypertrophic obstructive cardiomyopathy
ICP	Intracranial pressure
IDA	Iron deficiency anaemia
IDDM	Insulin-dependent diabetes mellitus
Ig	Immunoglobulin
IM	Intramuscular
INR	International normalized ratio (prothrombin ratio)
IPPV	Intermittent positive pressure ventilation
ITP	Idiopathic thrombocytopenic purpura
ITU	Intensive therapy unit
iu/IU	International unit
IV	Intravenous
IVI	Intravenous infusion
IVC	Inferior vena cava
IVU	Intravenous urography
JAMA	*Journal of the American Medical Association*
JVP	Jugular venous pressure
KCCT	Kaolin cephalin clotting time
L	Left
l	Litre(s)
LBBB	Left bundle branch block
LDH	Lactate dehydrogenase
LFT	Liver function test
LH	Luteinizing hormone
LIF	Left iliac fossa
LMN	Lower motor neurone
LP	Lumbar puncture
LUQ	Left upper quadrant
LVF	Left ventricular failure
LVH	Left ventricular hypertrophy
MCV	Mean cell volume
mg	Milligram(s)
MI	Myocardial infarction
mmHg	Millimetres of mercury
MND	Motor neurone disease
MS	Multiple sclerosis
MSU	Midstream urine
NB	*Nota bene* (note well)
NBM	Nil by mouth
ND	Notifiable disease
NEJM	*New England Journal of Medicine*
NG(T)	Nasogastric (tube)
NR	Normal range (= reference interval)
NSAIDs	Non-steroidal anti-inflammatory drugs

MEDICAL ABBREVIATIONS (cont'd)

N&V	Nausea and/or vomiting
OGS	Oxogenic steroids
ORh	Blood group O rhesus
P_aCO_2	Partial pressure of CO_2 in arterial blood
P_aO_2	Partial pressure of O_2 in arterial blood
PAN	polyarteritis nodosa
PBC	Primary biliary cirrhosis
PCV	Packed cell volume
PE	Pulmonary embolism
PEFR	Peak expiratory flow-rate
PID	Pelvic inflammatory disease
PIP	Proximal interphalangeal
PL	Prolactin
PND	Paroxysmal nocturnal dyspnoea
PR	*Per rectum* (rectal examination)
PPF	Purified plasma fraction (albumin)
PRL	Prolactin
PRN	*Pro re nata* (as required)
PRV	Polycythaemia rubra vera
PTH	Parathyroid hormone
PTT	Prothrombin time
R	Right
RA	Rheumatoid arthritis
RBBB	Right bundle branch block
RBC	Red blood cell
Rh	Rhesus
RhF	Rheumatic fever
RIF	Right iliac fossa
RUQ	Right upper quadrant
RVF	Right ventricular failure
SBE	Subacute bacterial endocarditis
SC	Subcutaneous
SD	Standard deviation
SE	Side-effects
SL	Sublingual
SLE	Systemic lupus erythematosus
SR	Slow release
SVC	Superior vena cava
SXR	Skull X-ray
$T\frac{1}{2}°$	Temperature
$t\frac{1}{2}$	Biological half-life
T_3	Triiodothyronine
T_4	Thyroxine
TB	Tuberculosis
TIA	Transient ischaemic attack
TRH	Thyroid releasing hormone
TPR	Temperature, pulse and respirations count
TSH	Thyroid stimulating hormone
u/U	Units
UC	Ulcerative colitis
U & E	Urea and electrolytes
UMN	Upper motor neuron
URT	Upper respiratory tract
URTI	Upper respiratory tract infection
UTI	Urinary tract infection
VDRL	Venereal diseases research laboratory
VMA	Vanilyl mandelic acid (HMMA)
VSD	Ventriculo-septal defect
WBC	White blood cell
WCC	White cell count
WR	Wasserman reaction
ZN	Ziehl–Neelsen

DAILY NUTRITIONAL REQUIREMENTS

Age	Calories (kcal)	Protein (g)	Calcium (g)	Iron (mg)	Thiamin (mg)	Riboflavin (mg)	Niacin (nicotinic acid equivalent) (mg)*	Vitamin B6 (mg)	Vitamin B12 (μg)	Folate (μg)	Vitamin C (mg)	Vitamin A (μg)	Vitamin D (μg)
0–3 months	120 per kg	3.0 per kg	0.6	5	0.2	0.4	3	0.2	0.3	50	25	350	8.5
4–9 months	110 per kg	3.0 per kg	0.8	5	0.2	0.4	4	0.3	0.4	50	25	350	7
10–12 months	100 per kg	2.5 per kg	1.0	7	0.3	0.4	5	0.4	0.4	50	25	350	7
1–3 years	1300	40	1.0	7	0.3	0.6	8	0.7	0.5	70	30	400	7
4–6 years	1700	40	1.0	8	0.7	0.8	11	0.9	0.8	100	30	400	—
7–10 years	2100	60	1.0	10	0.7	1.0	12	1.0	1.0	150	30	500	—
Men (70 kg)													
11–14 years	3100	85	1.4	15	0.9	1.2	15	1.2	1.2	200	35	600	—
15–18 years	3600	100	1.4	15	1.1	1.3	18	1.5	1.5	200	40	700	—
19–50 years	3200	70	0.8	10	1.0	1.3	17	1.4	1.5	200	40	700	†
50+ years	2550	70	0.8	10	0.9	1.3	16	1.4	1.5	200	40	700	†
Women (58 kg)													
11–14 years	2600	80	1.3	15	0.7	1.1	12	1.0	1.2	200	35	600	—
15–18 years	2460	75	1.3	15	0.8	1.1	14	1.2	1.5	200	40	600	—
19–50 years	2300	58	0.8	12	0.8	1.1	13	1.2	1.5	200	40	600	—
50+ years	1800	58	0.8	10	0.8	1.1	12	1.2	1.5	200	40	700	†
Pregnancy	2700	80	1.5	15	+0.1‡	+0.3	§	§	§	+100	+10	+100	10
Lactation													
0–4 months	3300	100	2.0	15	+0.2	+0.5	+2	§	§	+60	+30	+350	10
4+ months	3300	100	2.0	15	+0.2	+0.5	+2	§	§	+60	+30	+350	10

*Based on protein providing 14.7% of EAR for energy.
† After age 65 the daily RNI is 10 μg for men and women.
‡ For last trimester only.
§ No increment.

VITAMIN STATUS

Nutrient	Normal levels	Subnormal levels	Deficient levels
Vitamin A	20 µg/dl	10–19	<10
Thiamine	1.00–1.23 (ratio)	—	>1.23
Riboflavin	1.0–1.2 (ratio)	1.2–1.4	>1.4
Pyridoxine	1.15–1.19 (ratio)	—	>1.89
Niacin	—	—	—
Folate	6.0 µg/ml	3.0–5.9	<3.0
	160 µg/ml	140–159	<140
Vitamin B12	>160 ng/l	100–159	<100

FAT CONTENT OF FOODSTUFFS

	Total fat (%)	Saturates (%)	Monounsaturates (%)	Polyunsaturates (%)
Whole milk	7.5	11.9	5.8	1.3
Low fat milk	1.4	2.0	1.0	0.3
Cheese	6.1	9.7	4.6	1.4
Total milk/milk products	16.9	26.5	13.0	3.6
Carcass meat and poultry	12.8	12.4	15.2	7.8
Other meat and meat products	13.1	13.1	15.6	7.9
Total meat/meat products	25.9	25.5	30.8	15.7
Fish	1.6	0.9	1.6	3.1
Eggs	2.1	1.5	2.4	1.4
Butter	6.0	10.1	4.0	1.2
Margarine	12.2	8.3	12.9	22.1
Low fat and dairy spreads	4.1	3.8	4.9	3.6
Vegetable and salad oils	6.7	1.7	8.0	16.8
Total fats and oils	32.6	27.4	34.1	46.5
Vegetables	3.8	2.5	3.3	8.6
Fruit	1.6	1.0	1.7	2.7
Cakes, pastries, biscuits	8.0	9.5	7.7	5.4
Bread, breakfast cereals	3.0	1.5	1.6	5.5
Total cereals	13.2	12.8	11.2	13.7
Other foods and drinks	2.3	1.8	1.8	4.6
Total all foods (g/day)	84.9	33.7	31.5	13.8

FOOD TABLES

100g uncooked portion	Calories (kcal)	Water (g)	Protein (g)	Fat (g)	Carbohydrate Fibre (g)	Carbohydrate Total (g)
Vegetables						
Artichokes	29	90	2.7	0.2	1.9	5.8
Asparagus	22	93	2.0	0.2	0.8	4.0
Beans — kidney	335	12	21.3	1.6	4.0	61.5
— French	40	89	2.4	0.2	1.4	7.8
Beetroot	42	88	1.6	0.1	0.9	9.5
Broccoli	29	90	3.3	0.2	1.3	5.5
Brussels sprouts	48	85	4.6	0.5	1.2	8.7
Cabbage	25	92	1.4	0.2	1.0	5.7
Carrots — fresh	41	89	1.1	0.2	1.0	9.0
— canned	30	91	0.6	0.5	0.6	6.5
Cauliflower	26	92	2.4	0.2	0.9	5.0
Cucumber	13	96	0.8	0.1	0.6	3.0
Garlic	130	64	5.3	0.2	—	29.0
Leeks	44	88	2.0	0.3	1.3	9.4
Lettuce	15	95	1.4	0.2	0.6	2.8
Onions	46	87	1.5	0.2	0.8	10.3
Parsley	50	84	3.7	1.0	1.8	9.0
Parsnips	76	79	1.5	0.5	2.2	18.0
Peas — fresh	96	75	6.8	0.4	2.2	17.0
— dried	340	10	24.5	1.0	4.4	62.0
— canned	68	82	3.5	0.4	1.3	12.7
Potatoes	82	78	2.0	0.1	0.4	19.0
Spinach	20	93	2.3	0.3	0.7	3.2
Tomatoes	19	94	1.0	0.3	0.6	4.0
Tomato juice	19	94	1.0	0.2	—	4.3
Turnips	33	91	1.1	0.2	1.1	7.2
Watercress	18	94	1.7	0.3	0.5	3.2
Fish						
Caviare	295	36	33.5	17.0	—	—
Cod	74	83	16.0	0.4	—	—
Crab — canned	102	77	17.0	2.9	—	1.3
Eel — smoked	336	50	18.8	27.5	—	0.8
Haddock	80	81	18.2	0.1	—	—
Halibut	125	75	18.8	5.2	—	—
Herring	245	63	17.0	18.7	—	—
Mackerel	186	68	18.8	12.0	—	—
Oysters	67	83	9.0	1.2	—	4.9
Pike	90	80	18.3	1.2	—	—
Salmon — tinned	175	67	20.0	9.5	—	—
— fresh	206	66	19.8	13.6	—	—
Sardines	335	47	21.1	27.1	—	1.0
Shrimps	97	78	18.6	2.2	—	—
Trout	100	78	19.2	2.1	—	—
Fruit						
Apples	58	84	0.3	0.4	0.9	15.0
Apple juice	48	87	0.1	—	—	12.9
Apricots — fresh	50	85	0.9	0.2	0.6	13.0
Bananas	89	75	1.2	0.2	0.5	23.0
Cherries — fresh	61	83	1.1	0.4	0.5	14.7
Currants — black	62	82	1.0	0.1	3.2	16.2

FOOD TABLES (cont'd)

100g uncooked portion	Calories (kcal)	Water (g)	Protein (g)	Fat (g)	Carbohydrate Fibre (g)	Carbohydrate Total (g)
Dates — dried	280	20	2.2	0.6	2.4	76.0
Figs — dried	255	24	4.0	1.2	3.4	68.5
Gooseberries	38	89	0.8	0.2	1.2	9.6
Grapefruit	39	89	0.6	0.2	0.5	9.8
Grapes	66	82	0.8	0.4	4.3	16.5
Lemons	32	89	0.9	0.6	0.9	8.8
Melons — water	28	92	0.5	0.2	0.4	6.9
Oranges	45	87	0.9	0.2	0.8	11.2
Orange juice	48	86	0.6	0.1	0.1	12.9
Peaches	46	87	0.8	0.1	0.6	11.7
Pears	60	83	0.5	0.4	1.5	15.7
Pineapple	47	87	0.4	0.2	0.5	12.0
Plums	51	86	0.7	0.2	0.5	12.7
Prunes — dried	65	24	2.3	0.6	1.6	71.5
Raisins	65	24	2.3	0.5	1.8	71.0
Raspberries	57	84	1.2	0.4	2.8	13.9
Strawberries	37	90	0.8	0.5	1.2	8.2
Dairy produce						
Butter	716	17	0.6	82.0	—	0.7
Cheese — English	395	37	25.0	32.2	—	2.0
— cream	335	51	14.5	30.5	—	1.9
— cottage	86	79	17.3	0.6	—	1.8
Cream	290	64	2.2	30.5	—	2.9
Eggs	160	74	12.8	11.5	—	0.7
Egg powder	600	5	47.0	43.2	—	2.5
Milk — fresh, cows'	65	88	3.3	3.7	—	4.6
— condensed, sweet	320	27	8.0	8.4	—	54.8
— evaporated	140	74	7.0	7.9	—	9.9
— whole, dried	490	4	25.9	26.7	—	38.0
Bread, cereals						
Bread — white	244	35	9.2	1.2	0.2	52.5
— wholemeal	240	36	9.3	2.6	1.5	49.0
Cornflakes	383	4	8.1	0.4	0.6	85.0
Flour — white	360	12	10.5	1.0	0.3	76.0
— wheat	329	12.6	12.1	2.1	2.1	71.5
Rice — cooked	120	71	2.5	0.1	0.1	26.1
Semolina	359	13.1	10.3	0.8	—	76.0
Spaghetti	374	9	12.7	1.4	0.4	76.5
Tapioca — dry	360	12	0.6	0.2	0.1	86.5
Meat						
Bacon	620	20	9.1	64.0	—	—
Beef — corned	218	60	25.0	12.0	—	—
— roast	315	51	24.0	24.0	—	—
Chicken — roasters	200	66	20.3	12.5	—	—
Ham — boiled	270	57	19.5	20.5	—	—
Lamb — roast	272	56	24.0	19.0	—	—
L. chop — cooked	420	40	24.0	34.5	—	—
Pork loin — cooked	330	50	23.0	26.0	—	—

FOOD TABLES (cont'd)

100g uncooked portion	Calories (kcal)	Water (g)	Protein (g)	Fat (g)	Carbohydrate Fibre (g)	Carbohydrate Total (g)
Sausage — beef	284	49	13.8	18.5	—	15.8
— pork	337	51	8.8	28.8	—	9.7
Duck	322	54	16.0	28.0	—	—
Turkey	270	58	20.0	20.2	—	0.4
Veal — cooked	230	59	28.0	12.0	—	—
Miscellaneous						
Beer	44	90	0.6	4.0	—	4.0
Cocoa powder	298	6	20.0	24.5	—	43.6
Coconut — fresh	350	48	4.2	34.0	3.3	12.9
Cod liver oil	900	—	—	99.9	—	—
Coffee	5	98.5	0.3	0.1	—	0.8
Chocolate — plain	470	1.5	2.0	29.8	1.4	62.8
— milk	500	1	6.0	33.5	0.5	55.8
Honey	292	20	0.3	—	—	79.5
Mayonnaise	710	16	1.5	78.0	—	3.0
Peanuts — roasted	560	3	27.0	44.2	3.3	23.6
Sugar — white	382	trace	—	—	—	99.5
Tea	2	99	0.1	—	—	0.4
Whisky	250	—	—	35.0	—	—

1 kcal = 4.2 kJ (1000 kcal = 4200 kJ = 4.2 MJ). 1 lb = 453.6 g; 1 oz = 28.35 g.
1 fl oz = 28. 41 ml.

CONSTITUENTS OF HUMAN, ARTIFICIAL AND COWS' MILK

Constituent	Unit	Human milk	Highly modified baby milk	Modified baby milk	Cows' milk	Soy feed
Energy	k/100 ml	290	275	275	275	247
	kcal/100 ml	70	66	66	66	60
Protein	g/100 ml	1.1	1.5	1.9	3.5	2.0
Casein	%	40	40	80	82	0
Whey	%	60	60	20	18	0
Carbohydrate	g/100 ml	7.4	7.3	7.3	4.9	6.7
Fat	g/100 ml	4.2	3.6	3.4	3.7	3.0
Vegetable oil	—	—	**	**	—	***,**
Minerals						
Calcium	mg/l	35	54	85	117	55
Sodium	mg/l	15	18	25	50	30
Iron	mg/l	0.08	0.5	0.5	0.05	0.06

moderate amount * large amount

WEIGHT CONVERSION TABLE (STONES AND POUNDS TO KILOGRAMS)

Stones	Pounds													
	0	1	2	3	4	5	6	7	8	9	10	11	12	13
0		0.45	0.91	1.36	1.81	2.27	2.72	3.18	3.63	4.08	4.54	4.98	5.44	5.89
1	6.35	6.80	7.26	7.71	8.16	8.62	9.07	9.53	9.98	10.43	10.89	11.33	11.79	12.24
2	12.70	13.15	13.61	14.06	14.51	14.97	15.42	15.88	16.33	16.78	17.24	17.68	18.12	18.59
3	19.05	19.50	19.96	20.41	20.86	21.32	21.77	22.23	22.68	23.13	23.59	24.03	24.49	24.94
4	25.40	25.85	26.31	26.76	27.21	27.67	28.12	28.58	29.03	29.48	29.94	30.38	30.84	31.29
5	31.75	32.20	32.66	33.11	33.56	34.02	34.47	34.93	35.38	35.83	36.29	36.73	37.19	37.64
6	38.10	38.55	39.01	39.46	39.91	40.37	40.82	41.28	41.73	42.18	42.64	43.08	43.54	43.99
7	44.45	44.90	45.36	45.81	46.26	46.72	47.17	47.63	48.08	48.53	48.99	49.43	49.89	50.34
8	50.80	51.25	51.71	52.16	52.61	53.07	53.52	53.98	54.43	54.88	55.34	55.78	56.24	56.69
9	57.15	57.60	58.06	58.51	58.96	59.42	59.87	60.33	60.78	61.23	61.69	62.13	62.59	63.04
10	63.50	63.95	64.41	64.86	65.31	65.77	66.22	66.68	67.13	67.58	68.04	68.48	68.94	69.39
11	69.85	70.30	70.76	71.21	71.66	72.12	72.57	73.03	73.48	73.93	74.39	74.83	75.39	75.74
12	76.20	76.65	77.11	77.56	78.01	78.47	78.92	79.38	79.83	80.28	80.74	81.18	81.64	82.09
13	82.55	83.00	83.46	83.91	84.36	84.82	85.27	85.73	86.18	86.63	86.99	87.53	87.99	88.44
14	88.90	89.35	89.81	90.26	90.71	91.17	91.62	92.08	92.53	92.98	93.44	93.88	94.34	94.79
15	95.25	95.70	96.16	96.61	97.06	97.52	97.97	98.43	98.88	99.33	99.79	100.23	100.69	101.14
16	101.60	102.05	102.51	102.96	103.41	103.87	104.32	104.78	105.23	105.68	106.14	106.58	107.04	107.49
17	107.95	108.40	108.86	109.31	109.76	110.22	110.67	111.13	111.58	112.03	112.49	112.93	113.39	113.84
18	114.30	114.75	115.21	115.66	116.11	116.57	117.02	117.48	117.93	118.38	118.84	119.28	119.74	120.19

BACTERIAL STAINS

Method
(1) Add aqueous methyl violet 0.5% for one minute. (2) Wash. Cover with Gram's iodine for one minute. (3) Wash. Decolorize with alcohol/acetone for 30 to 60 seconds (until blue coloration disappears). (4) Wash and counterstain neutral red. (5) Wash and dry

Gram	
Positive	Negative
Cocci	
Pneumococcus	Neisseria catarrhalis
Staphylococcus	Neisseria gonorrhoeae
Streptococcus	Neisseria meningitidis
Rods	
Actinomyces	Bordetella pertussis
Bacillus anthracis	Brucella
Clostridium botulinus	Escherichia coli
Clostridium tetani	Haemophilus influenzae
Clostridium welchii	Klebsiella
Corynebacterium diphtheriae	Pasteurella pestis
Diphtheroids	Proteus
Mycobacterium tuberculosis	Pseudomonas aeruginosa
	Salmonellae, Shigellae
	Vibrio cholerae

EQUIVALENT DEGREES IN FAHRENHEIT AND CELSIUS $(°F - 32) \times \frac{5}{9} = °C$

The degree Celsius is identical in value to the degree Centigrade. A temperature interval or difference of 1°C is equivalent to 1 kelvin (K)

°F	°C	°F	°C	°F	°C
32 – 0		96 – 35.6		111 – 43.9	
50 – 10		97 – 36.1		112 – 44.4	
55 – 12.8		98 – 36.7		113 – 45	
60 – 15.6		98.4 – 36.9		114 – 45.6	
65 – 18.3		99 – 37.2		115 – 46.1	
68 – 20		100 – 37.8		116 – 46.7	
86 – 30		101 – 38.3		117 – 47.2	
87 – 30.6		102 – 38.9		118 – 47.8	
88 – 31.1		103 – 39.4		119 – 48.3	
89 – 31.7		104 – 40		120 – 48.9	
90 – 32.2		105 – 40.6		121 – 49.4	
91 – 32.8		106 – 41.1		122 – 50	
92 – 33.3		107 – 41.7		140 – 60	
93 – 33.9		108 – 42.2		158 – 70	
94 – 34.4		109 – 42.8		176 – 80	
95 – 35		110 – 43.3		212 – 100	

	°F	°C
Freezing	32	0
Boiling	212	100
Normal body temperature	98.4	36.9
Temperature of baths		
Cold	50–55	10–13
Tepid	70–90	21–32
Warm	90–100	32–38
Hot	100–105	38–40.5

SYSTÈME INTERNATIONAL BASE UNITS

Quantity	SI unit	Symbol
Length	Metre	m
Mass	Kilogram	kg
Time	Second	s
Electric current	Ampere	A
Thermodynamic temperature	Kelvin	K
Luminous intensity	Candela	cd
Amount of substance	Mole	mol

FRACTIONS AND MULTIPLES OF BASIC OR DERIVED SI UNITS

Prefix	Symbol	Multiple or fraction (using indices)	Value
Tera	T	10^{12}	1 000 000 000 000
Giga	G	10^9	1 000 000 000
Mega	M	10^6	1 000 000
Kilo	k	10^3	1000
Hecto	h	10^2	100
Deca	da	10^1	10
Deci	d	10^{-1}	0.1
Centi	c	10^{-2}	0.01
Milli	m	10^{-3}	0.001
Micro	μ	10^{-6}	0.000 001
Nano	n	10^{-9}	0.000 000 001
Pico	p	10^{-12}	0.000 000 000 001
Femto	f	10^{-15}	0.000 000 000 000 001
Atto	a	10^{-18}	0.000 000 000 000 000 001

The most widely used prefixes are kilo, milli and micro.
NB: $10^{-1} = 0.1 = 1/10$, $10^{-2} = 0.01 = 1/100$, $10^{-3} = 0.001 = 1/1000$, etc.
Indices should not be used when stating doses.

MEASUREMENTS IN COMMON USE

Mass		Volume	
pg	Picogram	fl	Femtolitre
ng	Nanogram	pl	Picolitre
μg	Microgram	nl	Nanolitre
mg	Milligram	μl	Microlitre
g	Gram	ml	Millilitre
kg	Kilogram	l	Litre
Time		Amount of substance	
s	Second	pmol	Picomole
ks	Kiloseconds	nmol	Nanomole
1 ks	16.67 minutes	μmol	Micromole
d	Day (24 hours)	mmol	Millimole

Blood gas measurements
1 kPa = 7.5007 mmHg; 1 mmHg = 133.32 Pa
(High pressure gas cylinders: 1 bar = 100 kPa = 14.5 psi)